Handbook of
Manual Muscle Testing

Handbook of
Manual Muscle Testing

EDITORS

Nancy C. Cutter, M.D.

Assistant Professor
Department of Rehabilitation Medicine
University of Colorado Health Sciences Center
and
Denver Veteran's Affairs Medical Center
Denver, Colorado

C. George Kevorkian, M.D.

Vice Chair and Associate Professor
Department of Physical Medicine and Rehabilitation
Baylor College of Medicine
and
Chief of Physical Medicine Service
St. Luke's Episcopal Hospital
Houston, Texas

McGraw-Hill
Health Professions Division

New York St. Louis San Francisco Auckland Bogotá Caracas Lisbon London Madrid
Mexico City Milan Montreal New Delhi San Juan Singapore Sydney Tokyo Toronto

McGraw-Hill

A Division of The McGraw·Hill Companies

HANDBOOK OF MANUAL MUSCLE TESTING

1234567890 DOCDOC 99

ISBN 0-07-033150-2

This book was set in Times Roman by T. C. Systems, Inc.
The editors were Stephen Zollo and Steven Melvin;
the production supervisor was Richard Ruzycka;
the designer was Robert Freese.
The index was prepared by Jerry Ralya.
R. R. Donnelley and Sons, Inc., was the printer and binder.

Figures in Chaps. 3 to 11 that carry the line "Copyright © 1997, McGraw-Hill." were reprinted, with permission from Garrison, D: *Illustrated Skeletal Muscles Flash Cards: Origins, Insertions, Functions, Innervations.* New York: McGraw-Hill, 1997. All other line art in those chapters was drawn by Holly R. Fischer, MFA, medical illustrator.

Library of Congress Cataloging-in-Publication Data

Handbook of manual muscle testing / editors, Nancy C. Cutter and C.
  George Kevorkian.
      p.   cm.
    Includes index.
    ISBN 0–07–033150–2
      1. Applied kinesiology—Handbooks, manuals, etc.   2. Muscle
  strength—Testing—Handbooks, manuals, etc.   I. Cutter, Nancy C.
  II. Kevorkian, C. George (Charles George)
      [DNLM: 1. Muscles—innervation.   2. Muscles—physiology.
  3. Myography—methods.   WE   500   H236   1999]
  RZ251.A65H36   1999
  612.7′4′0287—dc21
  DNLM/DLC
  for Library of Congress   98–55697

CONTENTS

CONTRIBUTORS

Donna Jo Blake, M.D. [4]
Associate Professor
Department of Rehabilitation Medicine
University of Colorado Health Sciences Center
and
Denver Veteran's Affairs Medical Center
Denver, Colorado

Carol Bodenheimer, M.D. [5]
Assistant Professor and Residency Program Director
Department of Physical Medicine and Rehabilitation
Baylor College of Medicine
and
Houston Veteran's Affairs Medical Center
Houston, Texas

Nancy C. Cutter, M.D. [1, 2]
Assistant Professor
Department of Rehabilitation Medicine
University of Colorado Health Sciences Center
and
Denver Veteran's Affairs Medical Center
Denver, Colorado

Fae H. Garden, M.D. [5]
Associate Professor
Department of Physical Medicine and Rehabilitation
Baylor College of Medicine
and
Associate Chief of Physical Medicine Service
St. Luke's Episcopal Hospital
Houston, Texas

Richard Gray, M.D., M.S. [10]
Associate Professor
Department of Physical Medicine and Rehabilitation
University of Arkansas for Medical Science
and
Assistant Chief for Clinical Affairs

Numbers in brackets refer to chapters written or cowritten by the contributors.

Physical Medicine and Rehabilitation Service
Central Arkansas Veterans Healthcare System
Little Rock, Arkansas

Cliff A. Gronseth, M.D. [6]
Assistant Professor
Department of Rehabilitation Medicine
University of Colorado Health Sciences Center
Denver, Colorado

Sally Ann Holmes, M.D. [9]
Assistant Professor
Department of Physical Medicine and Rehabilitation
Baylor College of Medicine
and
Assistant Chief
Spinal Cord Injury Service
Houston Veteran's Affairs Medical Center
Houston, Texas

Deanna M. Janora, M.D. [8]
Assistant Professor
University of Medicine and Dentistry of New Jersey
School of Osteopathic Medicine
Stratford, New Jersey

C. George Kevorkian, M.D. [1, 2]
Vice Chair and Associate Professor
Department of Physical Medicine and Rehabilitation
Baylor College of Medicine
and
Chief of Physical Medicine Service
St. Luke's Episcopal Hospital
Houston, Texas

Shelley A. Killen, M.D. [3]
Assistant Professor
Department of Physical Medicine and Rehabilitation
Medical College of Ohio
Toledo, Ohio

Dennis J. Matthews, M.D. [11]
Chairman and Associate Professor
Department of Rehabilitation Medicine
University of Colorado Health Sciences Center
and
Chairman, Department of Pediatric Physical Medicine and
    Rehabilitation
Children's Hospital
Denver, Colorado

Julie T. Miller, D.O. [3]
The Toledo Hospital
Toledo, Ohio

Scott Nadler, D.O. [7]
Assistant Professor
Department of Physical Medicine and Rehabilitation
University of Medicine and Dentistry of New Jersey
New Jersey Medical School
Newark, New Jersey

Todd Stitik, M.D. [7]
Assistant Professor
Department of Physical Medicine and Rehabilitation
University of Medicine and Dentistry of New Jersey
New Jersey Medical School
Newark, New Jersey

Marianne Sturr, M.S., D.O. [8]
Ability Rehabilitation Association
Salisbury, Maryland

Pamela E. Wilson, M.D. [11]
Clinical Professor
Children's Hospital
Denver, Colorado

PREFACE

The authors intend that readers of this handbook will achieve two worthwhile goals:

I. To learn the prerequisite "Basic Science" of muscle function so as to perform accurate and precise muscle testing. The reader must therefore gain and synthesize a significant knowledge level of

- Muscle innervation extending from nerve root to peripheral nerve. Helpful diagrams of dermatome levels and charts of myotomes are found throughout this text on a regional basis.
- Muscle origin and insertion; this is listed under each individual muscle.
- Muscle action in both an open and closed chain dynamic.
- Muscle agonists (synergists) and antagonists as no muscle acts alone in a musculoskeletal vacuum.

II. To master the practical "how to" of muscle testing and to apply this information in a clinical context.

To assist the reader we have incorporated photographs of desired examination techniques with specific instructions for the patient and tester. To further aid in developing "clinical savvy," significant clinical pearls and pitfalls of the muscle testing examination have been incorporated. A series of probing questions accompany each chapter and should further challenge the reader, who is urged to use these questions as a self-testing mechanism. Comprehensive appendices may be found at the end of the handbook.

The reader is cautioned that this handbook is not a substitute for a detailed anatomic or kinesiologic textbook. It should be used instead as a practical learning guide to the art and science of muscle testing.

Several chapters, by the unique nature of their topic material, deviate from the standard format of this text, but adhere to its basic principles and philosophy, containing both narrative text and relevant practical information on muscle testing. Throughout this handbook, various muscles have been omitted (Appendix 9). Reasons for omission include: clinical insignificance, extreme difficulty in isolation and/or testing, and lack of utility in establishing a diagnosis, treatment plan, and/or prognosis.

ACKNOWLEDGMENTS

Many fine friends and stalwart individuals supported the authors in the completion of this text. We are greatly in debt to them and offer the following tribute.

Julianna Woods, Jean Barnhill, Sarah Lenore Melanson, and Kimberly Hubbard were unselfish of their time and performed their secretarial duties above and beyond the call of normal office duty. Martin Kondreck was a pillar of strength, skill, and devotion in his performance as the volunteer photographer of this text. Those "low body fat," well-muscled models, Drs. Allison Fall, Robert Andrews, Cyril Bohachevsky, as well as Patrice Kennedy, P. T. and Michael Cutter not only were highly photogenic but not the least bit "camera shy." Our partners, Drs. Leigh Anderson, Fae H. Garden, Dan D. Scott, and Donna Jo Blake showed almost inhuman patience with us and readily pitched in to advise and help when needed. Virginia Clore, without having any formal background in biological sciences, showed her versatility by creating some of the illustrations used. Lastly to Michael and Jessica Cutter and Virginia Clore for being such a wonderful, patient, and loving family.

Handbook of
Manual Muscle Testing

CHAPTER 1

WHY MUSCLE TEST?

C. George Kevorkian and Nancy C. Cutter

The art and science of muscle isolation (if only partial) and testing provide the erudition and knowledge not otherwise available in today's technologically focused health care environment. Muscle testing, a critical and yet often overlooked component of the physical examination, can aid in precisely localizing a lesion in the peripheral nervous system. Knowledge of muscle function is imperative in many therapeutic interventions. Accurate muscle testing may influence a surgical decision. Prior to surgical transposition, one must be certain that remaining muscles can assume the function of the transposed muscle. Muscles rarely perform one single action. Instead they perform groups of actions which overlap with functions of other muscles. If muscle is lost, each component of its function may be compensated for by other muscles with duplicate functions. The therapeutic exercise program developed by a therapist or trainer is based on strengths and weaknesses identified by muscle testing. The results of muscle testing translate into potential function, which may determine whether a person can return to independent living or may need assistance.

GUIDELINES TO MUSCLE TESTING

Accurate muscle testing is achieved through proper subject positioning, appropriate maneuvers, and correct application of resistance. Below are suggested guidelines:

- Position the subject in the proper anti-gravity (grades 3 to 5) or gravity-eliminated (grades 0 to 2) position.
- Always compare passive to active range of motion (to achieve a grade of 3 to 5, the muscle must move through the entire "available" range).
- Body parts must be held firm and stable in order to prevent substitution.
- The patient must be comfortable, pain-free, and distraction-free.
- Stabilize appropriate parts of body so as to ensure an accurate muscle test. This may be provided by the exam plinth (table), other body muscles, or the examiner.
- Test position and movement patterns must be standardized.
- Apply pressure/force in the appropriate location and degree. Except when a longer lever is needed, this position is usually distally on the segment to where muscle insertion occurs. Pressure should be applied slowly, very gently, and gradually so as to accurately gauge true muscle strength. The examiner should then progress to the maximum resistance tolerable. It is never advisable to commence muscle testing while applying full

force. Naturally, the muscle tested and the patient's age, size, strength, and neuromusculoskeletal condition will influence the examiner. The application of force is usually made at the END of range in one-joint muscles and at midrange in two-joint muscles. Resistance should, if possible, be applied in the "line of pull" of the individual muscle(s).

PITFALLS

Pitfalls specific to the testing of any particular muscle are liberally sprinkled throughout this text. We list below pitfalls of a more generic nature of which the examiner must always be aware. (We assume the examiner has done his/her homework and is aware of basic anatomy and kinesiology.)

- Not isolating individual muscles with similar functions, that is, testing a muscle group rather than an individual muscle. This includes one-joint and two-joint muscles with similar function.
- Drawing conclusions regarding a patient's muscle strength when the examination was done in certain suboptimal circumstances:
  - The patient is sedated.
  - The patient is in significant pain.
  - The patient cannot be positioned properly.
  - Cultural or language barriers exist.
  - The patient has significant spasticity or hypertonicity.
  - Not considering both the gravity and gravity-eliminated position of the patient's muscles.
- Not being aware of basic substitution patterns which can exist in any given muscle test.
- "Overgrading" a muscle by applying pressure when the patient is unable to achieve the full available range of motion. It is possible for a weakened muscle to take resistance in a lengthened position despite being unable to achieve true full range of motion. Simply, the patient may not even have a muscle grade of 3 but can tolerate resistance in a lengthened position and an inexperienced tester might assign a grade greater than 3.
- "Undergrading" a muscle by not being aware of the effects of muscle contracture on range of motion. Thus, the muscle may appear to have not achieved full range of motion, when in fact it has achieved full "available" range of motion.

GRADING OF MUSCLES

The authors advocate the use of the 0 to 5 grading scale with 0 representing no muscle activity and 5 normal activity. To a great extent, this widely used grading system is based on that described by Robert Lovett, M.D., earlier this century. Although this scale relies on some degree of judgment by the examiner as to the amount of force resisted by the patient, the use of gravity resistance applies some objectivity to this method. Because of the precise definitions for 0 to 3 scores, there is little tester-to-tester variability. Scores of 4 to 5 require some subjectivity and hence may create more variability between testers. It should be noted that in certain strong muscles such as the gastrocnemius and gluteus maximus, the muscle can be considerably weakened before weakness can be clinically detected. Therefore a weakened muscle often can withstand maximum resistance and still be given the score of "5."

As a general rule, the use of + and − with this scale is to be discouraged unless the various health professionals treating the patient are consistent in their understanding of these modifiers. In any health care setting, such extra gradations therefore could be allowable if a uniform methodology existed (e.g., a grade of 2− for a patient who could achieve just partial movement—but greater than a flicker—with gravity eliminated).

Grades	Terms	Description
5	Normal	Achieves full available range against gravity and able to maintain maximal resistance.
4	Good	Achieves full available range against gravity and able to maintain moderate resistance.
3	Fair	Achieves full available range against gravity only. Cannot maintain against resistance.
2	Poor	Achieves full available range with gravity eliminated. Cannot perform this motion against gravity.
1	Trace	A visible or palpable contraction with no significant muscle movement.
0	Zero	No contraction seen or felt.

CHAPTER 2

BASIC KINESIOLOGY

C. George Kevorkian and Nancy C. Cutter

The majority of this book addresses *kinetics,* the forces that produce movement. First, however, a solid knowledge of *kinematics,* the geometry of motion, is necessary. In this chapter the authors will address the kinematic concepts of planes of motion, joint movements, and kinematic chains. Finally, types of muscle function, strengthening, and contractions will be addressed.

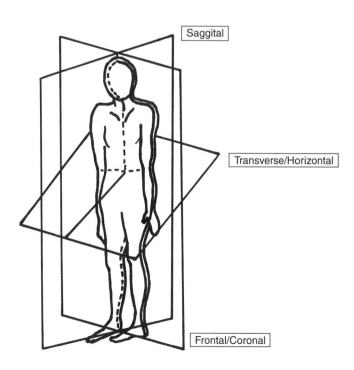

Saggital

Transverse/Horizontal

Frontal/Coronal

PLANES OF MOVEMENT

All body movements are defined in relation to three planes. Most natural body movements occur in a combination of these planes.

Sagittal

A vertical anteroposterior plane that divides the body into right and left halves. Examples of movement that occur in the sagittal plane include flexion and extension.

Frontal/Coronal

A vertical plane which traverses side to side and thus divides the body into front and back parts. Examples of movement that occur in the frontal plane are abduction and adduction.

Transverse/Horizontal

A horizontal plane that divides the body into upper and lower parts. Examples of movement that occur in the horizontal plane are internal and external rotation.

MOVEMENTS COMMON TO MOST JOINTS

Flexion

Movement of a joint in the sagittal plane so that the angle between the bones of the joint become smaller. Flexion of the hip, neck, trunk, head, and upper extremity occur in an anterior direction while that of the toes, foot, ankle, and knee are posteriorly directed.

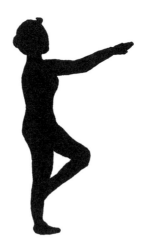

Extension

Movement of a joint in the sagittal plane so that straightening of the joint occurs and the angle of the sagittal plane becomes larger. The converse of flexion.

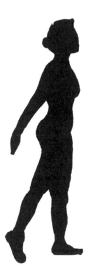

Abduction

Movement of a joint in the frontal/coronal plane so that the distal segment moves away from a defined line, usually the midsagittal plane of the body. Exceptions to the above include the toes, fingers, and thumb.

Toes

Movement away from the axial line that extends through the second digit.

Fingers

Movement away from the axial line that extends through the third digit.

Thumb

(see below)

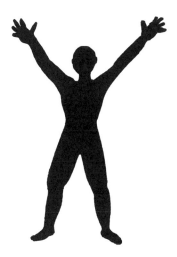

Adduction

Movement of a joint in the frontal/coronal plane so that the distal segment moves toward a defined line, usually the midsagittal plane. Exceptions to the above include the toes, fingers and thumb.

Toes

Movement toward the axial line that extends through the second digit.

Fingers

Movement toward the axial line that extends through the third digit.

Thumb

(see below)

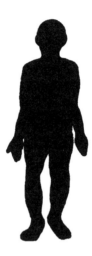

Internal Rotation (Medial Rotation)

Movement of a joint in the horizontal plane so any two points on separate segments on the anterior side come together. For example, during internal rotation of the shoulder, the forearm approximates the trunk.

External Rotation (Lateral Rotation)

Movement of a joint in the horizontal plane so any two points on separate segments on the posterior side come closer together. The converse of internal rotation.

Lateral Flexion

Movement in the coronal plane which refers to lateral movements of trunk, neck, and head (often combined with rotation).

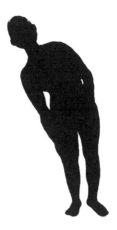

Supination

Movement of a joint toward the supine position. In the forearm supination occurs at the complex radioulnar joint resulting in turning the palm anteriorly. In
the foot, supination is a combination of inversion and adduction movements resulting in raising the longitudinal arch.

Pronation

Movement of a joint toward the prone position. In the forearm, pronation occurs at the complex radioulnar joint resulting in turning the palm posteriorly.
In the foot, pronation is a combination of eversion and abduction movements
resulting in a lowering of the longitudinal arch.

Circumduction

A combination of movements, usually flexion, extension, abduction, and adduction that result in a circular movement of the distal end of a limb.

Glide

Movement along the articulating surfaces of a joint such that the surfaces slide
along each other.

JOINTS WITH SPECIAL MOVEMENT
CONSIDERATIONS

SCAPULOTHORACIC JOINT

Adduction (Retraction)

Movement of the scapula toward the vertebral column.

Abduction (Protraction)

Movement of the scapula away from the vertebral column.

Elevation
Movement of the scapula cranially. This movement is represented by "shoulder shrugging."

Depression
Movement of the scapula caudally. This is the reverse of elevation and anterior tilt.

Upward Rotation (Lateral or External Rotation)
A rotational movement of the scapula so that the glenohumeral joint faces upward.

Downward Rotation (Medial or Internal Rotation)
A rotation movement of the scapula so that the glenohumeral joint faces downward.

Anterior Tilt
A combination of movements about the frontal axis so that the inferior angle of the scapula moves posteriorly and cranially and the coracoid process moves in an anterior and caudal direction.

GLENOHUMERAL JOINT

Shoulder Scaption
Arm elevation in the plane of the scapula as opposed to forward flexion and/or abduction. This is a highly functional movement.

Horizontal Abduction (Horizontal Extension)
With the shoulder elevated to 90 degrees in the transverse plane, the humerus is moved posterolaterally.

Horizontal Adduction (Horizontal Flexion)
With the shoulder elevated to 90 degrees in the transverse plane, the humerus is moved anteromedially.

CARPOMETACARPAL JOINT

Adduction
Movement perpendicular to the palm (going *towards* the palm).

Abduction
Movement perpendicular to the palm (going *away* from the palm).

Extension
Movement in a radial direction in the plane of the palm.

Flexion
Movement in an ulnar direction primarily in the plane of the palm (some abduction necessary for full flexion).

Opposition
See below.

METACARPOPHALANGEAL AND INTERPHALANGEAL JOINT

Extension
Movement in a radial direction in the plane of the palm.

Flexion
Movement in an ulnar direction in the plane of the palm.

Opposition

Occurs as a combination of abduction and flexion with medial rotation of the carpometacarpal joint and flexion of the metacarpophalangeal joint. Full opposition of the thumb and little finger requires the palmar surfaces, not the tips, of the fingers to come into contact.

TYPES OF MUSCLE STRENGTHENING

Isometric (Equal *Length*)

Occurs when there is a static contraction of a muscle. There is no motion of the muscle as a result of the contraction as both ends of the muscle are fixed.

Isotonic (Equal *Tension*)

Occurs when there is constant muscle contraction with constantly applied tension. The term *isotonic* is technically a misnomer because equal tension is not really exerted throughout joint range of motion. Isotonic exercise can be subdivided into two components:

- Concentric: Loading of the muscle occurs when the muscle is shortening.
- Eccentric: Loading of the muscle occurs when the muscle is lengthening.

Isokinetic (Equal *Speed*)

Occurs when there is muscle exercise at a predetermined constant velocity of joint motion. Isokinetic strength technically is the maximal torque that can be developed at any given velocity of contraction. Isokinetic exercise is designed to allow maximal force production through full range of motion. (Special equipment is usually needed for this type of strengthening.)

TYPES OF MUSCLE FUNCTION

Agonist (Prime Mover)

The muscle primarily or most responsible for a given movement.

Antagonist

A muscle acting against the action of the agonist.

Stabilizer

A muscle whose actions are required to create a necessary mechanical advantage for the prime mover or agonist.

Synergist

A muscle that assists the prime mover or agonist in its function(s).

KINETIC CHAINS

Open Chain

Occurs when the terminal segment is free to move, such as when the hand is waved or the foot is moved during the swing phase of gait.

Closed Chain

Occurs when the terminal segment is fixed, such as during a chin-up or a squat.

CHAPTER 3

SHOULDER AND ARM AND UPPER BACK

Shelley A. Killen and Julie T. Miller

UPPER AND LOWER SUBSCAPULAR
16. Subscapularis

SUPRASCAPULAR
17. Supraspinatus
18. Infraspinatus

MUSCULOCUTANEOUS
19. Coracobrachialis
20. Biceps Brachii
21. Brachialis

RADIAL
21. Brachialis
22. Triceps Brachii and Anconeus

MUSCLES OMITTED
Subclavius

MUSCLE FUNCTION AT SPECIFIC JOINTS

Shoulder Flexion
Anterior deltoid
Coracobrachialis
Long head of biceps brachii
Pectoralis major (clavicular)

Shoulder Extension
Latissimus dorsi
Teres major
Posterior deltoid
Long head of triceps brachii
Pectoralis major (when the shoulder is flexed beyond 90 degrees)

Shoulder Abduction
Anterior deltoid (in combination with the posterior deltoid)
Middle deltoid
Supraspinatus
Biceps brachii (in combination with other abductors when the shoulder is abducted
beyond 90 degrees)

Shoulder Adduction
Latissimus dorsi
Teres major
Pectoralis major (clavicular)
Pectoralis major (sternal)
Coracobrachialis
Long head of triceps brachii

Shoulder Horizontal Adduction
Pectoralis major (clavicular)
Anterior deltoid
Coracobrachialis

Shoulder Horizontal Abduction
Posterior deltoid

Shoulder Internal Rotation
> Latissimus dorsi
> Teres major
> Pectoralis major (Clavicular)
> Anterior deltoid
> Subscapularis

Shoulder External Rotation
> Posterior deltoid
> Teres minor
> Infraspinatus

Elbow Flexion
> Biceps brachii
> Brachialis
> Brachioradialis
> Pronator teres
> Extensor carpi radialis longus
> Flexor carpi radialis
> Palmaris longus
> Flexor carpi ulnaris

Elbow Extension
> Triceps brachii
> Anconeus

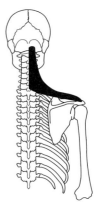

1. UPPER TRAPEZIUS

Origin
- External occipital protuberance
- Medial third of superior nuchal line of occipital bone
- Upper part of ligamentum nuchae
- C7 vertebrae spinous process

Insertion
- Posterior border of lateral third of clavicle
- Acromion process of scapula

Roots N/A

Trunk N/A

Cord N/A

Nerve
- Cranial nerve XI (Spinal accessory nerve)
- Ventral rami of C2-4 (Controversial, more likely a sensory contribution only)

Open Chain Actions
SOLO ACTION
- Scapular elevation (lateral angle)
- Scapular adduction
- Rotation of head to opposite side (unilateral)
- Lateral flexion of head to same side (unilateral)

COMBINED ACTION
- Scapular elevation with levator scapulae [5]
- Scapular adduction with rhomboids [4] / middle trapezius [2]
- Head and cervical extension bilaterally
- Scapular upward rotation with serratus anterior [6] and lower trapezius [3]

Closed Chain Action N/A

Synergists

Muscle	Nerve	Root
• Rhomboid major and minor [4]	Dorsal scapular	C5
• Middle trapezius [2]	Spinal accessory	CN XI, C2-4
• Levator scapulae [5]	Nerve to the levator scapulae; dorsal scapular	C3-5
• Serratus anterior [6]	Long thoracic	C5-7

Antagonists

Muscle	Nerve	Root
• Lower trapezius [3]	Spinal accessory	CN XI, C2-4
• Pectoralis minor [11]	Medial pectoral	C7-T1
• Subclavius	N. to subclavius	C5-6
• Pectoralis major (Sternal) [10]	Medial pectoral	C8-T1
• Serratus anterior [6]	Long thoracic	C5-7
• Latissimus dorsi [7]	Thoracodorsal	C6-8

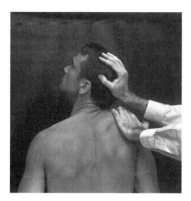

MUSCLE TESTING INSTRUCTIONS

Patient

Sitting with arms relaxed at sides. The patient raises the shoulder as high as possible and extends and rotates occiput towards the elevated shoulder.

Tester

The tester generates resistance downward on top of the shoulders and against the head in the direction of flexion anterolaterally.

Test

"Raise your shoulder up to the ceiling against my hand and try to touch the back of your head to your shoulder."

Pitfalls

N/A

CLINICAL PEARLS

1. Weakness of the trapezius [1,2,3] secondary to a lesion of the spinal accessory nerve often manifests itself as a characteristic winging of the scapula. This winging is made obvious by shoulder abduction and is sometimes termed lateral winging.
2. Tension of the costoclavicular ligament limits scapular elevation.
3. Unilateral contracture is often seen in torticollis.
4. Weakness interferes with the ability to abduct and flex the humerus above shoulder level.
5. This muscle is a common location of trigger points.

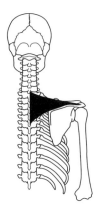

2. MIDDLE TRAPEZIUS

Origin
- Inferior part of ligamentum nuchae
- Spinous processes of seventh cervical and superior thoracic vertebrae (horizontal fibers of muscle)

Insertion
- Medial margin of acromion process of scapula
- Superior lip of posterior border of spine of the scapula

Roots N/A

Trunk N/A

Cord N/A

Nerve
- Cranial nerve XI (spinal accessory nerve)
- Ventral rami of C2-4 (controversial, more likely a sensory contribution only)

Open Chain Action
SOLO ACTION
- Scapular adduction (retraction)

COMBINED ACTION
- Scapular adduction with rhomboids [4] and lower trapezius [3]

Closed Chain Action N/A

Synergists

Muscle	Nerve	Root
• Rhomboid major and minor [4]	Dorsal scapular	C5
• Trapezius upper and lower [1,3]	Spinal accessory	CN XI, C2-4
• Serratus anterior [6]	Long thoracic	C5-7
• Levator scapulae [5]	Nerve to the levator scapulae, dorsal scapular	C3-5

Antagonists

Muscle	Nerve	Root
• Serratus anterior [6]	Long thoracic	C5-7
• Pectoralis major [9,10]	Medial and lateral pectoral	C5-T1
• Pectoralis minor [11]	Medial pectoral	C7-T1
• Lower trapezius [3]	Spinal accessory	CN XI, C2-4

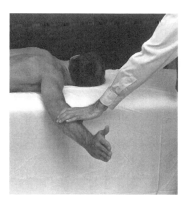

MUSCLE TESTING INSTRUCTIONS

Patient

Prone with the elbow extended and the shoulder abducted to 90 degrees and laterally rotated. The palm should be facing cranially and the shoulder girdle should *not* be elevated.

Tester

The tester generates pressure against the forearm in a downward direction toward the table.

Test

"With your palm up and your arm out straight from your side, push against my hand."

Pitfalls

If the arm is not laterally rotated, the fibers of the middle trapezius [2] are not being tested.

CLINICAL PEARLS

1. See Clinical Pearls of the upper trapezius [1], as applicable.

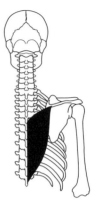

3. LOWER TRAPEZIUS

Origin
- Spinous processes of thoracic vertebrae T7-12 and corresponding supraspinal ligament

Insertion
- Via an aponeurosis sliding over the medial end of the spine of the scapula to a tubercle at the apex of the smooth triangular surface of the root of the scapula

Roots N/A

Trunk N/A

Cord N/A

Nerve
- Cranial nerve XI (spinal accessory nerve)
- Ventral rami of C2-4 (Controversial, more likely a sensory contribution only)

Open Chain Action
SOLO ACTION
- Scapular depression
- Scapular adduction
- Scapular upward rotation

COMBINED ACTION
- Scapular adduction with middle fibers of trapezius [2]
- Scapular upward rotation with serratus anterior [6] and upper trapezius [1]
- Shoulder depression with latissimus dorsi [7] and pectoralis minor [11]

Closed Chain Action N/A

Synergists

Muscle	Nerve	Root
• Middle trapezius [2]	Spinal accessory	CN XI, C2-4
• Upper trapezius [1]	Spinal accessory	CN XI, C2-4
• Serratus anterior [6]	Long thoracic	C5-7
• Pectoralis minor [11]	Medial pectoral	C7-T1
• Latissimus dorsi [7]	Thoracodorsal	C6-8

Antagonists

Muscle	Nerve	Root
• Upper trapezius [1]	Spinal accessory	CN XI, C2-4
• Levator scapulae [5]	Nerve to the levator scapulae; dorsal scapular	C3-5
• Rhomboid major and minor [4]	Dorsal scapular	C5
• Serratus anterior [6]	Long thoracic	C5-7

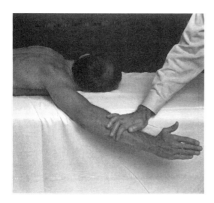

MUSCLE TESTING INSTRUCTIONS

Patient

The patient is lying prone with the arm placed diagonally overhead and the shoulder laterally rotated.

Tester

The tester generates pressure against the forearm downward toward the plinth.

Test

"With your arm diagonally upward and your palm facing upward, push against my hand."

Pitfalls

N/A

CLINICAL PEARLS

1. See Clinical Pearls of upper trapezius [1], as applicable.

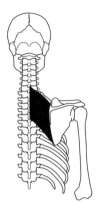

4. RHOMBOID MAJOR AND MINOR

Origin
- Major: Spinous processes of the second through the fifth thoracic vertebrae
- Minor: Ligamentum nuchae, spinous processes of seventh cervical and first thoracic vertebrae

Insertion
- Major: By fibrous attachment to medial border of scapula between spine and inferior angle.
- Minor: Medial border at the root of the spine of scapula.

Roots C5

Trunk N/A

Cord N/A

Nerve Dorsal scapular

Open Chain Action

SOLO ACTION
- Scapular adduction
- Scapular elevation
- Downward rotation of the scapula so that the glenoid cavity faces caudally

COMBINED ACTION
- Scapular adduction with levator scapulae and trapezius
- Scapular elevation with levator scapulae and upper trapezius
- Scapular downward rotation with the levator scapulae

Closed Chain Action Fixes the medial border of the scapula.

Synergists

Muscle	Nerve	Root
• Levator scapulae [5]	Nerve to the levator scapulae; dorsal scapular	C3-5
• Trapezius (all divisions) [1,2,3]	Spinal accessory	CN XI, C2-4

Antagonists

Muscle	Nerve	Root
• Pectoralis major and minor [9,10,11]	Lateral and medial pectoral	C5-T1
• Latissimus dorsi [7]	Thoracodorsal	C6-8
• Lower trapezius [3]	Spinal accessory	CN XI, C2-4
• Serratus anterior [6]	Long thoracic	C5-7

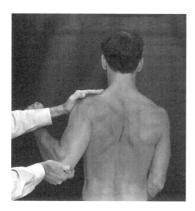

MUSCLE TESTING INSTRUCTIONS

Patient

Prone with elbow flexed, the ipsilateral humerus is adducted, slightly extended, and externally rotated. (For photography purposes, this picture was taken in a sitting position.)

Tester

Apply pressure with one hand against the patient's arm in the direction of abducting the scapula and rotating the inferior angle laterally; and against the patient's shoulder with the other hand in the direction of depression.

Test

"With your face down and turned toward me, bend your elbow and try to move your arm backwards."

Pitfalls

Do not allow the patient to force the head of the humerus downward against the table in an attempt to lift the arm. Both the arm and scapula should move together.

CLINICAL PEARLS

1. Strength of adduction and extension of the humerus is diminished by loss of rhomboid fixation of the scapula. Ordinary function of the arm is affected less by loss of rhomboids than by loss of either trapezius [1,2,3] or serratus anterior [6].
2. Weakness of this muscle may result in medial winging.
3. The dorsal scapular nerve comes directly off of the cervical nerve roots and *not* the brachial plexus.

5. LEVATOR SCAPULAE

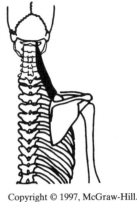

Origin
- Transverse processes of first four cervical vertebrae

Insertion
- Medial border of the scapula between superior angle and root of spine

Roots C3-5

Trunk N/A

Cord N/A

Nerve
- Nerve to the levator scapulae (C3-4)
- Some authors consider that the dorsal scapular (C5) gives off a twig to this muscle

Open Chain Action
SOLO ACTION
- Scapular elevation
- Downward rotation of the scapula so the glenoid cavity faces caudally
- Scapular retraction (adduction)

COMBINED ACTION
- Downward rotation of the scapula
- Scapular adduction
- Cervical spine extension

Closed Chain Action N/A

Synergists

Muscle	Nerve	Root
• Trapezius (all divisions) [1,2,3]	Spinal accessory	CN XI, C2-4
• Rhomboid major and minor [4]	Dorsal scapular	C5

Antagonists

Muscle	Nerve	Root
• Serratus anterior [6]	Long thoracic	C5-7
• Lower trapezius [3]	Spinal accessory	CN XI, C2-4
• Pectoralis minor [11]	Medial pectoral	C7-T1
• Subclavius	Nerve to subclavius	C5-6
• Pectoralis major (lower) [9,10]	Medial pectoral	C8-T1
• Latissimus dorsi [7]	Thoracodorsal	C6-8

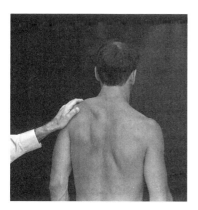

MUSCLE TESTING INSTRUCTIONS

Patient
Sitting with arms relaxed at sides, raise shoulders as high as possible.

Tester
The tester generates resistance downward on top of the shoulders.

Test
"Raise your shoulders up as high as you can and don't let me push them down."

Pitfalls
It is difficult to differentiate strength of the levator scapulae from that of the trapezius [1].

CLINICAL PEARLS

1. When there is weakness of the trapezius [1,2,3], there may be an excessive elevation of the superior angle of the scapula because of increased activity of the levator scapulae.
2. The levator scapulae [5] is a common site of trigger points.

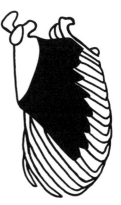

6. SERRATUS ANTERIOR

Origin
- Outer surfaces and superior borders of upper eight or nine ribs
- Aponeuroses covering intercostal muscles

Insertion
- Ventral surface of superior angle of scapula
- Ventral surface of vertebral border of scapula
- Lower 5 or 6 digitations converge and insert on ventral surface of inferior angle of scapula

Roots C5-7

Trunk N/A

Cord N/A

Nerve Long thoracic

Open Chain Action
SOLO ACTION
- Scapular abduction
- Upward rotation of the scapula so that the glenoid cavity faces cranially
- Holds the medial border of the scapula firmly against the thorax
- Scapular depression (lower fibers)
- Scapular elevation (upper fibers)

COMBINED ACTION
- Displaces the thorax posteriorly when the humerus is fixed in flexion
- Scapular protraction with the pectoralis minor [11]
- Scapular upward rotation with upper and lower trapezius [1,3]
- Scapular depression with pectoralis minor [11], pectoralis major [9,10], latissimus dorsi [7], subclavius, and lower trapezius [3]

Closed Chain Action N/A

Synergists

Muscle	Nerve	Root
• Trapezius (upper and lower) [1,3]	Spinal accessory	CN XI, C2-4
• Pectoralis minor [11]	Medial pectoral	C7-T1
• Latissimus dorsi [7]	Thoracodorsal	C6-8
• Subclavius	Nerve to subclavius	C5-6

Antagonists

Muscle	Nerve	Root
• Rhomboid major and minor [4]	Dorsal scapular	C5
• Middle trapezius [2]	Spinal accessory	CN XI, C2-4
• Levator scapulae [5]	Nerve to the levator scapulae; dorsal scapular	C3-5

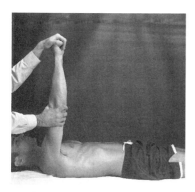

MUSCLE TESTING INSTRUCTIONS

Patient

Technique 1: Supine with the shoulder flexed to 90 degrees with slight abduction and with the elbow in extension. The patient moves the arm upward by abducting the scapula.

Technique 2: Standing with the patient's hands pressed against a wall with the shoulders in forward flexion to 80 to 90 degrees. The elbows should be locked in extension.

Tester

Technique 1: Resistance is given by grasping around the forearm and elbow. Pressure is downward and inward toward the table.

Technique 2: Observe the patient while he/she is pushing against the wall.

Test

Technique 1: "Hold your arm out straight from the table and try to lift it higher by moving your shoulder forward while I push down on it."

Technique 2: "Push against the wall."

Pitfalls

Movement of the scapula must be observed and the inferior angle palpated to ensure that there is no substitution.

CLINICAL PEARLS

1. Weakness of this muscle results in "winging" of the scapula, especially the inferior angle.
2. Serratus anterior [6] weakness makes it difficult to raise the arm in flexion or abduction.
3. Along with the ribs, the serratus anterior [6] forms the medial wall of the axilla.
4. The long thoracic nerve comes directly off of the cervical nerve roots and *not* the brachial plexus.

7. LATISSIMUS DORSI

Origin
- Posterior layer of lumbodorsal fascia by which it is attached to spines of the lower six thoracic, lumbar, and sacral vertebrae, supraspinal ligament, and to the posterior iliac crest
- External lip of iliac crest lateral to erector spinae
- Ribs 9-12
- Usually a few fibers from the inferior angle of scapula

Insertion
- Distal aspect of the intertubercular groove of the humerus

Roots C6-8

Trunk Upper, middle, and lower

Cord Posterior

Nerve Thoracodorsal

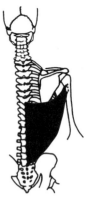

Open Chain Action
SOLO ACTION
- Shoulder internal rotation
- Shoulder adduction
- Shoulder extension
- Depression of shoulder girdle

COMBINED ACTION
- Lateral flexion of the trunk
- Hyperextension of the spine

Closed Chain Action
- Assists in tilting the pelvis anteriorly and laterally
- Accessory muscle of respiration
- In the "on hands and knees" position, contraction of this muscle combined with the teres major [8] rocks the torso forward

Synergists

Muscle	Nerve	Root
• Teres major [8]	Lower subscapular	C5-6
• Posterior deltoid [14]	Axillary	C5-6
• Triceps brachii (long head) [22]	Radial	C6-8
• Erector spinae	Dorsal primary divisions adjacent to spinal nerves	
• Anterior deltoid [12]	Axillary	C5-6
• Subscapularis [16]	Upper and lower subscapular	C5-6
• Pectoralis major [9,10]	Medial and lateral pectoral	C5-T1

Antagonists

Muscle	Nerve	Root
• Middle deltoid [13]	Axillary	C5-6
• Supraspinatus [17]	Suprascapular	C5-6
• Infraspinatus [18]	Suprascapular	C5-6
• Teres minor [15]	Axillary	C5-6
• Anterior deltoid [12]	Axillary	C5-6
• Coracobrachialis [19]	Musculocutaneous	C5-7
• Biceps brachii [20]	Musculocutaneous	C5-6
• Posterior deltoid [14]	Axillary	C5-6
• Pectoralis major (clavicular) [9]	Lateral pectoral	C5-7

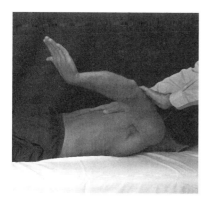

MUSCLE TESTING INSTRUCTIONS

Patient

Prone with the shoulder medially rotated and adducted with the palm up to prevent lateral rotation. The patient extends the shoulder through the range of motion.

Tester

The tester stabilizes the thorax. Resistance is given proximal to the elbow joint. Force is generated in a vector combination of abduction and minimal flexion of the arm.

Test

"Lying on your stomach, lift your arm straight up keeping your palm toward the ceiling."

Pitfalls

Do not allow flexion of the thoracic spine or abduction at the shoulder joint.

CLINICAL PEARLS

1. The latissimus dorsi [7] is a very important muscle for crutch walking or any activity that pulls the body toward the arm (rock climbing, pulling up on parallel bars).
2. The latissimus dorsi [7] is a major source of power for swimming, rowing, chopping movements.
3. Shortness of the latissimus dorsi [7] results in limitation of elevation of the arm in flexion or abduction. This situation is seen in scoliosis, kyphosis, or long-time crutch users.
4. The latissimus dorsi [7] is active in strong expiration (coughing and sneezing) and deep inspiration.

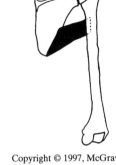

8. TERES MAJOR

Origin
- Dorsal surfaces of the inferior angle and lower third of the lateral border of the scapula
- Fibrous septa between this muscle and the teres minor [15] and infraspinatus [18]

Insertion
- Crest of lesser tubercle of the humerus (posterior to the latissimus dorsi [7])

Roots C5-6

Trunk Upper

Cord Posterior

Nerve Lower subscapular

Open Chain Action
SOLO ACTION
- Shoulder internal rotation
- Shoulder adduction
- Shoulder extension

COMBINED ACTION N/A

Closed Chain Action In the "on hands and knees" position, contraction of this muscle combined with the latissimus dorsi [7] rocks the torso forward.

Synergists

Muscle	Nerve	Root
• Latissimus dorsi [7]	Thoracodorsal	C6-8
• Posterior deltoid [14]	Axillary	C5-6
• Triceps brachii (long head) [22]	Radial	C6-8
• Pectoralis major [9,10]	Medial and lateral pectoral	C5-T1
• Subscapularis [16]	Upper and lower subscapular	C5-6
• Anterior deltoid [12]	Axillary	C5-6

Antagonists

Muscle	Nerve	Root
• Middle deltoid [13]	Axillary	C5-6
• Supraspinatus [17]	Suprascapular	C5-6
• Infraspinatus [18]	Suprascapular	C5-6
• Teres minor [15]	Axillary	C5-6
• Coracobrachialis [19]	Musculocutaneous	C5-7
• Biceps brachii [20]	Musculocutaneous	C5-6
• Anterior deltoid [12]	Axillary	C5-6
• Posterior deltoid [14]	Axillary	C5-6
• Pectoralis major (clavicular) [9]	Lateral pectoral	C5-7

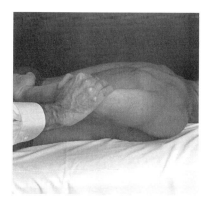

MUSCLE TESTING INSTRUCTIONS

Patient

Prone with the arm extended, adducted and medially rotated with the hand resting on the small of the back.

Tester

The tester generates resistance against the arm proximal to the elbow in a vector of abduction and flexion.

Test

"Put your arm behind your back, resting your hand on your hip and push your arm against my hand."

Pitfalls

N/A

CLINICAL PEARLS

1. Scapular movements (lateral rotation) which accompany shoulder flexion and abduction are influenced by shortness of the teres major [8] and subscapularlis [16].
2. The teres major [8] forms the inferior border of the quadrilateral space.
3. The teres major [8] is sometimes called "the little latissimus" because it performs the same movements as the latissimus dorsi [8].

9. PECTORALIS MAJOR (CLAVICULAR)

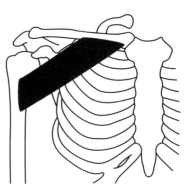

Origin
- Anterior surface of the sternal half of the clavicle

Insertion
- Crest of the greater tubercle of the humerus (anterior and caudal)

Roots C5-7

Trunk Upper and middle

Cord Lateral

Nerve Lateral pectoral

Open Chain Action

SOLO ACTION
- Shoulder flexion
- Shoulder internal rotation
- Shoulder horizontal adduction

COMBINED ACTION N/A

Closed Chain Action
- Assists in elevating the thorax in forced inspiration
- Assists in supporting the weight of the body in crutch-walking or in parallel bar ambulation

Synergists

Muscle	Nerve	Root
• Pectoralis major (sternal) [10]	Medial pectoral	C8- T1
• Subscapularis [16]	Upper and lower subscapular	C5-6
• Latissimus dorsi [7]	Thoracodorsal	C6-8
• Teres major [8]	Lower subscapular	C5-6
• Anterior deltoid [12]	Axillary	C5-6
• Coracobrachialis [19]	Musculocutaneous	C5-7
• Pectoralis minor [11]	Medial pectoral	C7-T1
• Serratus anterior [6]	Long thoracic	C5-7
• Biceps brachii [20]	Musculocutaneous	C5-6
• Middle deltoid [13]	Axillary	C5-6

Antagonists

Muscle	Nerve	Root
• Latissimus dorsi {7]	Thoracodorsal	C6-8
• Teres major [8]	Lower subscapular	C5-6
• Posterior deltoid [14]	Axillary	C5-6
• Infraspinatus [18]	Suprascapular	C5-6
• Triceps brachii (long head) [22]	Radial	C6-8
• Teres minor [15]	Axillary	C5-6
• Supraspinatus [17]	Suprascapular	C5-6
• Middle deltoid [13]	Axillary	C5-6

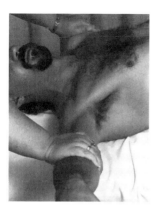

MUSCLE TESTING INSTRUCTIONS

Patient

Supine with the shoulder in 60 to 90 degrees of abduction and elbow flexed. Patient is then asked to horizontally adduct the shoulder.

Tester

The tester generates resistance proximal to the wrist in a downward and outward direction.

Test

"Move your arm up and in across your chest."

Pitfalls

If the elbow flexors are weak, provide resistance proximal to the elbow.

CLINICAL PEARLS

1. This muscle is important in crutch walking and ambulation in parallel bars.
2. The pectoralis major [9] can be ruptured in arm wrestling by a sudden forceful medial rotation and adduction of the shoulder.
3. The patient may be unable to touch the opposite shoulder if weakened.

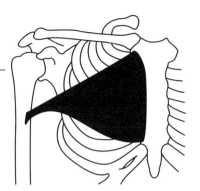

10. PECTORALIS MAJOR (STERNAL)

Origin
- Anterior surface of the sternum, and the cartilages of the first six or seven ribs
- Aponeurosis of the external oblique

Insertion
- Crest of the greater tubercle of the humerus. (Lower fibers twist on themselves and are more posterior and cranial.)

Roots C8-T1

Trunk Lower

Cord Medial

Nerve Medial pectoral

Open Chain Action
SOLO ACTION
- Depresses the shoulder girdle
- Adducts the arm toward the opposite iliac crest

COMBINED ACTION N/A

Closed Chain Action
- Assists in elevating the thorax in forced inspiration
- Assists in supporting the weight of the body in crutch-walking or in parallel bar gait
- Assists in drawing the trunk upward and forward in climbing

Synergists

Muscle	Nerve	Root
• Pectoralis major (clavicular) [9]	Lateral pectoral	C5-7
• Posterior deltoid [14]	Axillary	C5-6
• Latissimus dorsi [7]	Thoracodorsal	C6-8
• Teres major [8]	Lower subscapular	C5-6
• Triceps brachii (long head) [22]	Radial	C6-8
• Pectoralis minor [11]	Medial pectoral	C8-T1

Antagonists

Muscle	Nerve	Root
• Supraspinatus [17]	Suprascapular	C5-6
• Deltoid [12,13,14]	Axillary	C5-6
• Trapezius [1,2,3]	Spinal accessory	CN XI, C2-4
• Serratus anterior [6]	Long thoracic	C5-7
• Levator scapulae [5]	Nerve to the levator scapulae, dorsal scapular	C3-5
• Rhomboid major and minor [4]	Dorsal scapular	C5

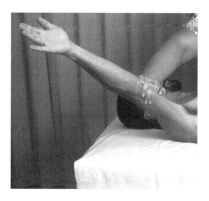

MUSCLE TESTING INSTRUCTIONS

Patient

Supine with the shoulders in 120 degrees abduction with elbow flexed. The patient moves the arm down and in, across the body.

Tester

The tester generates resistance proximal to the elbow in an up and outward vector.

Test

"Move your arm down and in across your body."

Pitfalls

If the elbow flexors are weak, provide resistance proximal to the elbow.

CLINICAL PEARLS

1. This muscle is important in crutch walking and in ambulation in the parallel bars.
2. Chopping or striking movements are difficult if this muscle is weak.
3. If this muscle is weak, it will be difficult to hold any large or heavy objects in both hands at or near waist level.
4. This muscle forms the anterior wall of the axilla.
5. Absence of the sternal portion of the pectoralis major [10] results in no significant disability, but the anterior axillary fold is absent and the nipple is lower.

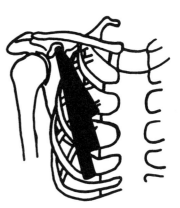

11. PECTORALIS MINOR

Origin
- Superior margins and outer surfaces of ribs 3 to 5 near the cartilages
- Fascia overlying the corresponding intercostal muscles

Insertion
- Medial border, superior surface of the coracoid process of the scapula

Roots C7-T1

Trunk Middle and lower

Cord Medial and lateral

Nerve
- Medial pectoral

Open Chain Action
SOLO ACTION
- Depresses the shoulder
- Scapular downward rotation
- Scapular protraction

COMBINED ACTION
- Elevation of ribs in forced inspiration

Closed Chain Action Assists in forced inspiration when the scapula is fixed by the levator scapulae.

Synergists

Muscle	Nerve	Root
• Pectoralis major [9,10]	Medial and lateral pectoral	C5-T1
• Lower trapezius [3]	Spinal accessory	CN XI, C2-4
• Serratus anterior [6]	Long thoracic	C5-7
• Latissimus dorsi [7]	Thoracodorsal	C6-8
• Levator scapulae [5]	Nerve to levator scapulae: dorsal scapular	C3-5
• Rhomboid major and minor [4]	Dorsal scapular	C5
• Middle trapezius [2]	Spinal accessory	CN XI, C2-4

Antagonists

Muscle	Nerve	Root
• Trapezius [1,2,3]	Spinal accessory	CN XI, C2-4
• Levator scapulae [5]	Nerve to levator scapulae, dorsal scapular	C3-5
• Rhomboid major and minor [4]	Dorsal scapular	C5
• Serratus anterior [6]	Long thoracic	C5-7
• Latissimus dorsi [7]	Thoracodorsal	C6-8

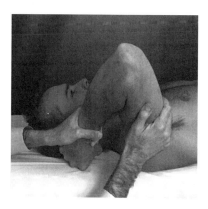

MUSCLE TESTING INSTRUCTIONS

Patient
Supine with the arm at the side. The shoulder girdle is lifted from the table.

Tester
The tester generates resistance against the anterior aspect of the shoulder, downward toward the table.

Test
"Raise your shoulder off the table and don't let me push it down."

Pitfalls
The patient should not be allowed to exert downward pressure on the hand to force the shoulder forward. It is essential to keep the elbow and hand off the table when testing.

CLINICAL PEARLS

1. Arm extension may be weak if the pectoralis minor [11] is weak because of decreased scapular stabilization.
2. If this muscle is tight, arm pain may result secondary to impingement on the cords of the brachial plexus or axillary vessels (one version of the controversial "thoracic outlet syndrome").
3. Contracture may result in decreased shoulder flexion.
4. The pectoralis minor [11] forms the anterior wall of the axilla.
5. The pectoralis minor [11] can act as a shoulder protractor.
6. Occasionally, fibers from a communicating branch of the lateral pectoral nerve may innervate the pectoralis minor [11]. However, this is rare.

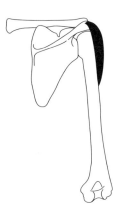

12. ANTERIOR DELTOID

Origin
- Anterior border, superior surface of the lateral third of the clavicle

Insertion
- Deltoid tuberosity of the humerus

Roots C5-6

Trunk Upper

Cord Posterior

Nerve Axillary

Open Chain Action
SOLO ACTION
- Shoulder horizontal adduction
- Shoulder flexion
- Internal rotation
- Shoulder scaption (arm elevation in the plane of the scapula: see Clinical Pearls)

COMBINED ACTION
- Shoulder abduction

Closed Chain Action In the "on hands and knees" position, the anterior deltoid rocks the torso backward.

Synergists

Muscle	Nerve	Root
Middle and posterior deltoid [13,14]	Axillary	C5-6
Supraspinatus [17]	Suprascapular	C5-6
Coracobrachialis [19]	Musculocutaneous	C5-7
Pectoralis major [9,10]	Lateral and medial pectoral	C5-T1
Biceps brachii [20]	Musculocutaneous	C5-6
Subscapularis [16]	Upper and lower subscapular	C5-6

Antagonists

Muscle	Nerve	Root
Posterior deltoid [14]	Axillary	C5-6
Latissimus dorsi [7]	Thoracodorsal	C6-8
Teres major [8]	Lower subscapular	C5-6
Infraspinatus [18]	Suprascapular	C5-6
Teres minor [15]	Axillary	C5-6
Triceps brachii (long head) [22]	Radial	C6-8

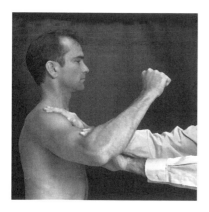

MUSCLE TESTING INSTRUCTIONS

Patient
Technique 1: Sitting with the shoulder abducted in minimal flexion and lateral rotation.
Technique 2: Supine with the shoulder abducted in minimal flexion and internal rotation.

Tester
Technique 1: The tester generates resistance to the volar and medial aspect of the arm, in the vector of adduction and minimal extension.
Technique 2: The tester places one hand under the patient's wrist to make sure it does not press on the chest and resistance is generated against the anterior surface of the arm just above the elbow, in the direction of adduction toward the side of the body.

Test
"Place your arm diagonally out from your body with your palm upward. Don't let me push it down."

Pitfalls
N/A

CLINICAL PEARLS

1. Shoulder scaption (arm elevated in the plane of the scapula) is the position more frequently used for function than either forward flexion or abduction.

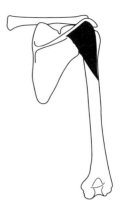

13. MIDDLE DELTOID

Origin
- Lateral margin and superior surface of the acromion of the scapula

Insertion
- Deltoid tuberosity of the humerus

Roots C5-6

Trunk Upper

Cord Posterior

Nerve Axillary

Open Chain Action
SOLO ACTION
- Shoulder abduction

COMBINED ACTION
- Shoulder scaption
- Shoulder flexion

Closed Chain Action N/A

Synergists

Muscle	Nerve	Root
• Supraspinatus [17]	Suprascapular	C5-6
• Anterior deltoid [12]	Axillary	C5-6
• Posterior deltoid [14]	Axillary	C5-6

Antagonists

Muscle	Nerve	Root
• Latissimus dorsi [7]	Thoracodorsal	C6-8
• Teres major [8]	Lower subscapular	C5-6
• Triceps brachii (long head) [22]	Radial	C6-8
• Coracobrachialis [19]	Musculocutaneous	C5-7

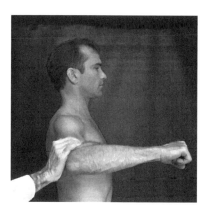

MUSCLE TESTING INSTRUCTIONS

Patient
Sitting with the arm abducted to 90 degrees with slight elbow flexion.

Tester
The tester generates resistance just proximal to the elbow in a downward direction.

Test
"Lift your arm out to the side to shoulder level and don't let me push it down."

Pitfalls
Do not let the patient substitute using the biceps brachii [20] by externally rotating the shoulder.

CLINICAL PEARLS

1. When testing the middle deltoid [13], do not allow shoulder elevation or lateral flexion of the trunk to the opposite side as these create an illusion of abduction.

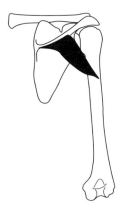

14. POSTERIOR DELTOID

Origin
- Inferior lip of the posterior border of the spine of scapula

Insertion
- Deltoid tuberosity of the humerus

Roots C5-6

Trunk Upper

Cord Posterior

Nerve Axillary

Open Chain Action

SOLO ACTION
- Shoulder extension
- Shoulder horizontal abduction
- External rotation

COMBINED ACTION
- Shoulder abduction

Closed Chain Action In the "on hands and knees position," the posterior deltoid rocks the torso forward.

Synergists

Muscle	Nerve	Root
• Latissimus dorsi [7]	Thoracodorsal	C6-8
• Teres major [8]	Lower subscapular	C5-6
• Long head triceps brachii [22]	Radial	C6-8
• Infraspinatus [18]	Suprascapular	C5-6
• Teres minor [15]	Axillary	C5-6

Antagonists

Muscle	Nerve	Root
• Anterior deltoid [12]	Axillary	C5-6
• Pectoralis major [9,10]	Medial and lateral pectoral	C5-T1
• Coracobrachialis [19]	Musculocutaneous	C5-7
• Biceps brachii [20]	Musculocutaneous	C5-6
• Subscapularis [16]	Upper and lower subscapular	C5-6
• Latissimus dorsi [7]	Thoracodorsal	C6-8
• Teres major [8]	Lower subscapular	C5-6

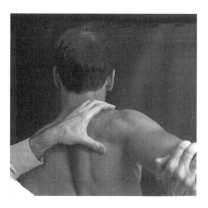

MUSCLE TESTING INSTRUCTIONS

Patient
Sitting with the shoulder abducted with minimal extension and internal rotation.

Tester
The tester generates resistance to the dorsolateral aspect of the arm, proximal to the elbow, in the vector of adduction and minimal flexion.

Test
"Push your arm back towards me."

Pitfalls
If the elbow is not maintained in flexion, the long head of the triceps brachii [22] will, in effect, substitute for the posterior deltoid.

CLINICAL PEARLS

1. When testing this muscle, if the scapular muscles are weak, the examiner must stabilize the scapula manually to avoid scapular protraction.

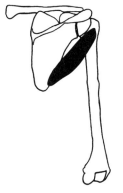

15. TERES MINOR

Origin
- Upper two-thirds of the dorsal surface of the axillary border of the scapula
- Fascia separating it from the teres major [8] and the infraspinatus [18]

Insertion
- Lowest facet of the greater tubercle of the humerus (below the insertion of the infraspinatus [18])

Roots C5-6

Trunk Upper

Cord Posterior

Nerve Axillary

Open Chain Action
SOLO ACTION
- Shoulder external rotation

COMBINED ACTION
- Stabilizes humeral head in the glenoid cavity during shoulder movements
- Shoulder adduction

Closed Chain Action N/A

Synergists

Muscle	Nerve	Root
• Infraspinatus [18]	Suprascapular	C5-6
• Posterior deltoid [14]	Axillary	C5-6

Antagonists

Muscle	Nerve	Root
• Subscapularis [16]	Upper and lower subscapular	C5-6
• Pectoralis major [9,10]	Medial and lateral pectoral	C5-T1
• Latissimus dorsi [7]	Thoracodorsal	C6-8
• Teres major [8]	Lower subscapular	C5-6
• Anterior deltoid [12]	Axillary	C5-6

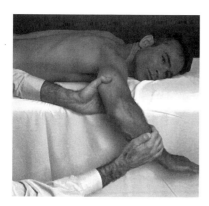

MUSCLE TESTING INSTRUCTIONS

Patient
Prone with the shoulder abducted to 90 degrees. The arm must be supported by the plinth and the forearm must be allowed to move freely. The patient externally rotates the shoulder so that the forearm becomes level with the plinth.

Tester
The tester generates gentle resistance at the wrist while the other hand supports the elbow.

Test
"Bring your forearm even with the plinth and stop me from pushing it down."

Pitfalls
Supination may be mistaken for shoulder external rotation if the teres minor [15] is weak. Resistance should be given gradually and slowly to avoid injury secondary to inherent instability of the shoulder joint.

CLINICAL PEARLS

1. The teres minor [15] is a rotator cuff muscle.
2. The teres minor [15] forms the superior border of quadrilateral space.
3. The teres minor [15] and the infraspinatus [18] are virtually inseparable in muscle testing.

16. SUBSCAPULARIS

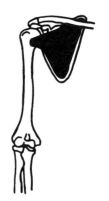

Origin
- Subscapular fossa and the groove along the axillary margin of the scapula

Insertion
- Lesser tubercle of the humerus and anterior capsule of the glenohumeral joint

Roots C5-6

Trunk Upper

Cord Posterior

Nerve Upper and lower subscapular

Copyright © 1997, McGraw-Hill.

Open Chain Action

SOLO ACTION
- Shoulder internal rotation

COMBINED ACTION
- Stabilizes the humeral head in the glenoid cavity during shoulder movements

Closed Chain Action N/A

Synergists

Muscle	Nerve	Root
• Pectoralis major [9,10]	Medial and lateral pectoral	C5-T1
• Latissimus dorsi [7]	Thoracodorsal	C6-8
• Teres major [8]	Lower subscapular	C5-6
• Anterior deltoid [12]	Axillary	C5-6

Antagonists

Muscle	Nerve	Root
• Infraspinatus [18]	Suprascapular	C5-6
• Teres minor [15]	Axillary	C5-6
• Posterior deltoid [14]	Axillary	C5-6

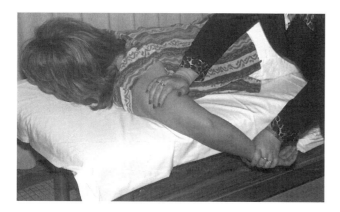

MUSCLE TESTING INSTRUCTIONS

Patient

The patient is supine with the shoulder abducted to 90 degrees. The hand is by the head. The patient moves the forearm forward and down.

Tester

The tester generates resistance on the volar aspect of the forearm in a backward and downward position.

Test

"Move your forearm towards me and don't let me push it back."

Pitfalls

The patient may try to substitute by pronating the forearm, a movement which can be mistaken for shoulder internal rotation.

CLINICAL PEARLS

1. Internal rotation of the shoulder is a much stronger movement than external rotation secondary to greater muscle mass.
2. By depressing the humerus, the subscapularis [16] keeps the humeral head in the glenoid fossa.
3. The subscapularis [16] is a rotator cuff muscle.
4. With the scapula, this muscle forms the posterior wall of the axilla.
5. It is very difficult to isolate this muscle from the other very strong shoulder internal rotators.

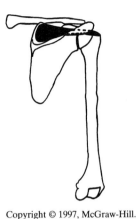

17. SUPRASPINATUS

Origin
- Medial two-thirds of the supraspinous fossa of the scapula and the fascia covering the supraspinatus

Insertion
- Superior facet of the greater tubercle of the humerus

Roots C5-6

Trunk Upper

Cord N/A

Nerve Suprascapular

Open Chain Action
SOLO ACTION
- Shoulder abduction

COMBINED ACTION
- Shoulder scaption
- Stabilizes the humeral head in the glenoid cavity during shoulder movements
- Shoulder external rotation

Closed Chain Action N/A

Synergists

Muscle	Nerve	Root
• Deltoid [12,13,14]	Axillary	C5-6

Antagonists

Muscle	Nerve	Root
• Teres major [8]	Lower subscapular	C5-6
• Latissimus dorsi [7]	Thoracodorsal	C6-8
• Pectoralis major [9,10]	Medial and lateral pectoral	C5-T1

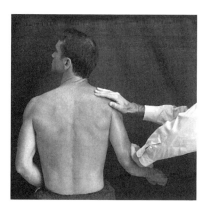

MUSCLE TESTING INSTRUCTIONS

Patient

Standing or sitting with the arm resting comfortably by the side, the patient's head is rotated ipsilaterally and extended. The shoulder is abducted to 90 degrees. Another option is to do the testing with the arm at the side and for the tester to palpate the muscle at the beginning of abduction.

Tester

The tester generates resistance proximal to elbow in an adduction vector.

Test

"Keep your arm up at shoulder level and stop me from pushing it down." Or "Try to push your arm out against my hand."

Pitfalls

It is clinically difficult to distinguish this muscle from the middle deltoid [13] as they essentially fire simultaneously. It is important to palpate this muscle to see if it is active. When testing this muscle, shoulder external rotation should not be allowed as the patient may be substituting the biceps brachii [20]. In addition, movements such as shoulder elevation, external rotation, or lateral flexion of the trunk should not be permitted to occur because these movements also lead to either substitution or false abduction.

CLINICAL PEARLS

1. Rupture of the supraspinatus [17] tendon decreases shoulder joint stability.
2. The supraspinatus [17] is the muscle most often involved in "shoulder impingement syndrome."
3. The supraspinatus [17] is a rotator cuff muscle.
4. The nerve supply of this muscle comes off of the upper trunk before any cords of the brachial plexus are formed.

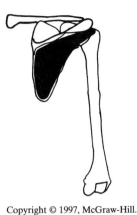

18. INFRASPINATUS

Origin
- Medial two-thirds of the infraspinous fossa of the scapula and the fascia covering the infraspinatus

Insertion
- Middle facet of the greater tubercle of the humerus

Roots C5-6

Trunk Upper

Cord N/A

Nerve Suprascapular

Open Chain Action
SOLO ACTION
- Shoulder external rotation

COMBINED ACTION
- Stabilizes the humeral head in the glenoid cavity during shoulder movements

Closed Chain Action N/A

Synergists

Muscle	Nerve	Root
• Teres minor [15]	Axillary	C5-6
• Posterior deltoid [14]	Axillary	C5-6

Antagonists

Muscle	Nerve	Root
• Subscapularis [16]	Upper and lower subscapular	C5-6
• Pectoralis major [9,10]	Medial and lateral pectoral	C5-T1
• Latissimus dorsi [7]	Thoracodorsal	C6-8
• Teres major [8]	Lower subscapular	C5-6
• Anterior deltoid [12]	Axillary	C5-6

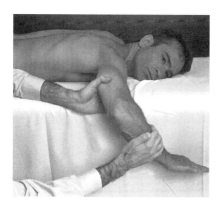

MUSCLE TESTING INSTRUCTIONS

Patient
Prone with the shoulder abducted to 90 degrees. The arm must supported by the plinth and the forearm must be allowed to move freely. The patient externally rotates the shoulder so that the forearm becomes level with the plinth.

Tester
The tester generates gentle resistance at the wrist while the other hand supports the elbow.

Test
"Bring your forearm even with the plinth and stop me from pushing it down."

Pitfalls
Supination may be mistaken for external rotation if the infraspinatus is weak. Resistance should be given gradually and slowly to avoid injury secondary to inherent instability of the shoulder joint.

CLINICAL PEARLS

1. The infraspinatus [18] is a rotator cuff muscle.
2. The infraspinatus [18] and teres minor [15] are virtually inseparable in muscle testing.
3. The nerve supply to this muscle comes off of the upper trunk before any cords of the brachial plexus are formed.

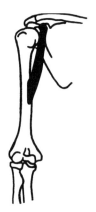

19. CORACOBRACHIALIS

Origin
- Apex of the coracoid process of the scapula

Insertion
- Medial surface of the mid-humerus, opposite the deltoid tuberosity

Roots C5-7

Trunk Upper and middle

Cord Lateral

Nerve Musculocutaneous

Open Chain Action

SOLO ACTION
- Shoulder flexion
- Shoulder adduction
- Shoulder horizontal adduction

COMBINED ACTION N/A

Closed Chain Action N/A

Synergists

Muscle	Nerve	Root
• Anterior deltoid [12]	Axillary	C5-6
• Pectoralis major (clavicular) [9]	Lateral pectoral	C5-7
• Biceps brachii [20]	Musculocutaneous	C5-6
• Latissimus dorsi [7]	Thoracodorsal	C6-8
• Teres major [8]	Lower subscapular	C5-6

Antagonists

Muscle	Nerve	Root
• Latissimus dorsi [7]	Thoracodorsal	C6-8
• Posterior deltoid [13]	Axillary	C5-6
• Teres major [8]	Lower subscapular	C5-6
• Triceps brachii (long head) [22]	Radial	C6-8
• Middle deltoid [13]	Axillary	C5-6
• Supraspinatus [17]	Suprascapular	C5-6

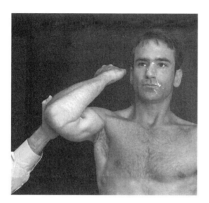

MUSCLE TESTING INSTRUCTIONS

Patient

Sitting or supine with the shoulder flexed and in minimal external rotation, the elbow is at maximal flexion and supination.

Tester

The tester generates resistance against the volar and medial aspect of the distal humerus in the vector of extension and minimal abduction.

Test

"Bend your elbow with your palm up and raise your arm to shoulder level. Don't let me push it down."

Pitfalls

The arm should stay in the neutral position so the patient does not substitute the biceps brachii [20] for flexion. Avoid shoulder elevation so the patient cannot substitute the upper trapezius [1]. Avoid horizontal adduction so the patient cannot substitute the pectoralis major [9,10]. The patient should not be allowed to lean backwards to assist with flexion.

CLINICAL PEARLS

1. The coracobrachialis [19] does not cross the elbow joint and hence has no action there.
2. The musculocutaneous nerve may be trapped as it enters the coracobrachialis [19] muscle. In these rare cases, this muscle usually receives its normal innervation, but the nerve supply to the biceps brachii [20] and brachialis [21] may be affected.

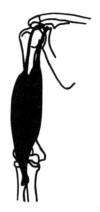

20. BICEPS BRACHII

Origin
- Short head: Apex of the coracoid process of the scapula
- Long head: Supraglenoid tubercle of the scapula

Insertion
- Radial tuberosity and the aponeurosis of the biceps brachii

Roots C5-6

Trunk Upper

Cord Lateral

Nerve Musculocutaneous

Open Chain Action
SOLO ACTION
- Elbow flexion
- Forearm supination
- Shoulder flexion (weak)

COMBINED ACTION
- Shoulder abduction (involvement usually occurs after 90 degrees)
- During deltoid activity, stabilizes and depresses the humeral head in the glenoid

Closed Chain Action During a "chin-up," this muscle contributes to elevation of the body.

Synergists

Muscle	Nerve	Root
• Brachialis [21]	Musculocutaneous	C5-7
• Brachioradialis [23]	Radial	C5-6
• Supinator [24]	Radial	C5-6
• Anterior deltoid [12]	Axillary	C5-6
• Coracobrachialis [19]	Musculocutaneous	C5-7
• Pectoralis major (clavicular) [9]	Lateral pectoral	C5-7
• Flexor carpi radialis [33]	Median	C6-8
• Flexor carpi ulnaris [50]	Ulnar	C8-T1
• Pronator teres [32]	Median	C6-7
• Extensor carpi radialis longus and brevis [25]	Radial	C6-7

Antagonists

Muscle	Nerve	Root
• Triceps brachii and anconeus [22]	Radial	C6-8
• Pronator teres [32]	Median	C6-7
• Pronator quadratus [38]	Median	C7-T1
• Latissimus dorsi [7]	Thoracodorsal	C6-8
• Posterior deltoid [14]	Axillary	C5-6

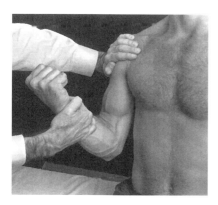

MUSCLE TESTING INSTRUCTIONS

Patient

The patient flexes the elbow with the forearm in supination.

Tester

The tester generates resistance over the volar forearm in an extension vector while stabilizing the shoulder.

Test

"Bend your elbow."

Pitfalls

The wrist flexors should remain relaxed during the test as they may assist in elbow flexion.

CLINICAL PEARLS

1. If there is a musculocutaneous nerve lesion, the forearm will pronate as it flexes because of the relatively unopposed activity of the brachioradialis [23] muscle.
2. Painless rupture of the long head of the biceps brachii [20] is often associated with increased age and lifting. This resembles a "Popeye" muscle.
3. Chin-ups done with the forearm pronated are usually more difficult because the biceps brachii [20] is at a mechanical disadvantage.

21. BRACHIALIS

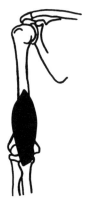

Origin
- Distal two-thirds of the anterior surface of the humerus and the intermuscular septa between the brachialis and the triceps brachii [22]

Insertion
- Tuberosity and coronoid process of ulna

Roots C5-7

Trunk Upper and middle

Cord Lateral and posterior

Nerve Musculocutaneous and radial

Open Chain Action
Solo Action
- Elbow flexion

Combined Action N/A

Closed Chain Action During a "chin-up," this muscle contributes to elevation of the body.

Synergists

Muscle	Nerve	Root
• Biceps brachii [20]	Musculocutaneous	C5-6
• Brachioradialis [23]	Radial	C5-6
• Flexor carpi radialis [33]	Median	C6-8
• Flexor carpi ulnaris [50]	Ulnar	C8-T1
• Pronator teres [32]	Median	C6-7
• Extensor carpi radialis longus and brevis [25]	Radial	C6-7

Antagonists

Muscle	Nerve	Root
• Triceps brachii and anconeus [22]	Radial	C6-8

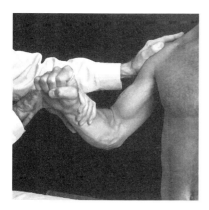

MUSCLE TESTING INSTRUCTIONS

Patient

Sitting or supine, the patient flexes the elbow with the forearm in pronation.

Tester

The tester generates resistance over the dorsal surface of the forearm proximal to the wrist in the direction of elbow extension while stabilizing the shoulder.

Test

"Bend your elbow with your palm downward and stop me from pulling it down."

Pitfalls

Wrist flexors and extensors should remain relaxed during testing as they may assist in elbow flexion.

CLINICAL PEARLS

1. The distal, lateral part of this muscle receives innervation from a branch off of the Radial nerve.
2. The brachialis [21] does not participate in supination or pronation of the forearm.
3. The brachialis [21] is considered a dually innervated muscle.

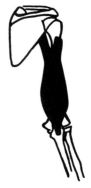

22. TRICEPS BRACHII AND ANCONEUS

Origin
- Long head: Infraglenoid tubercle of the scapula.
- Lateral head: Lateral and posterior surfaces of the proximal one-half of the body of the humerus and the lateral intermuscular septum.
- Medial head: Distal two-thirds of the medial and posterior surfaces of the humerus below the radial groove and from the medial intermuscular septum.
- Anconeus: Posterior surface of the lateral epicondyle of the humerus and dorsal aspect of the elbow joint capsule.

Copyright © 1997, McGraw-Hill.

Insertion
- Triceps: Posterior surface of the olecranon process of the ulna and the antebrachial fascia.
- Anconeus: Lateral side of the olecranon process and upper one-fourth of the posterior surface of the body of the ulna.

Roots C6-8

Trunk Upper, middle, and lower

Cord Posterior

Nerve Radial

Open Chain Action

SOLO ACTION
- Elbow extension
- Shoulder extension (long head)
- Shoulder adduction (long head)

COMBINED ACTION N/A

Closed Chain Action During a "push-up," the triceps brachii extends the elbow so as to elevate the body.

Synergists

Muscle	Nerve	Root
• Latissimus dorsi [7]	Thoracodorsal	C6-8
• Teres major [8]	Lower subscapular	C5-6
• Posterior deltoid [14]	Axillary	C5-6

Antagonists

Muscle	Nerve	Root
• Biceps brachii [20]	Musculocutaneous	C5-6
• Brachioradialis [22]	Radial	C5-6
• Brachialis [21]	Musculocutaneous	C5-7
• Flexor carpi radialis [33]	Median	C6-8
• Flexor carpi ulnaris [50]	Ulnar	C8- T1
• Pronator teres [32]	Median	C6-7
• Extensor carpi radialis longus and brevis [25]	Radial	C6-7

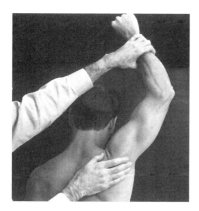

MUSCLE TESTING INSTRUCTIONS

Patient
Technique 1: Prone with the shoulder abducted to 90 degrees, the patient extends the elbow and then unlocks it (just less than total extension).
Technique 2: Supine with the shoulder abducted to 180 degrees, the patient extends the elbow and then unlocks it (just less than total extension).
Technique 3: Sitting with the shoulder abducted to 180 degrees, the patient extends the elbow and then unlocks it (just less than total extension).

Tester
The tester generates resistance against the forearm after the patient has fully extended the elbow joint.

Test
"Straighten your elbow all the way, unlock it, and stop me from bending it."

Pitfalls
N/A

CLINICAL PEARLS

1. Substitution for a weakened triceps brachii [22] can often be achieved by shoulder external rotation or horizontal adduction.
2. The long head of the triceps brachii [22] forms the medial side and the lateral head the lateral side of the quadrilateral space.
3. In fractures of the proximal humerus, the radial nerve is often injured. However, the branch of the radial nerve to the triceps brachii [22] is often spared because of its proximal location. In such cases, the distal muscles innervated by the radial nerve may be affected while the triceps brachii is spared.
4. Substitution for elbow extension in transfers can be achieved by placing the hand on a surface in a closed chain position and flexing the shoulder to lock the elbow. Thus, patients with absent triceps brachii [22] function (i.e., C6 tetraplegics) may still be able to transfer.

QUESTIONS

1. How would you clinically differentiate scapular winging caused by weakness of the serratus anterior [6] muscle from that caused by a weakened trapezius [1,2,3] muscle?
2. Name five internal rotators of the shoulder and their innervation.
3. Name at least six muscles which assist the biceps brachii [20] in elbow flexion.
4. What are the three major functions of the lower trapezius [3] muscle?
5. What is the "other" scapular protractor (in addition to the serratus anterior [6] muscle)?
6. What tendon is most commonly involved in impingement syndrome at the shoulder?
7. What two maneuvers does a tetraplegic spinal-cord injured person use for elbow extension in the absence of triceps brachii [22] function?
8. Define shoulder "scaption" and what two muscles perform this movement.
9. What tendon rupture results in a "Popeye" arm?
10. What is the ratio of movement of the glenohumeral joint to the scapula?

FOREARM AND HAND

Donna Jo Blake

37. Flexor digitorum profundus (and *median*)
41. Flexor pollicis brevis: Deep and superficial heads (and *median*)
42. Lumbricals (and *median*)

MUSCLES OMITTED
Extensor digiti minimi

MUSCLE FUNCTION AT SPECIFIC JOINTS

Forearm supination
Biceps brachii
Brachioradialis
Supinator

Forearm pronation
Brachioradialis
Pronator teres
Pronator quadratus
Flexor carpi radialis

Wrist extension
Extensor carpi radialis longus
Extensor carpi radialis brevis
Extensor carpi ulnaris
Extensor digitorium communis
Extensor indicis
Extensor digiti minimi
Extensor pollicis longus

Wrist flexion
Flexor carpi radialis
Flexor carpi ulnaris
Palmaris longus
Flexor digitorum profundus
Flexor digitorum superficialis
Flexor pollicis longus

Wrist ulnar deviation
Flexor carpi ulnaris
Extensor capri ulnaris

Wrist radial deviation
Flexor carpi radialis
Extensor carpi radialis longus
Extensor carpi radialis brevis
Extensor pollicis longus
Extensor pollicis brevis
Abductor pollicis longus

Metacarpophalangeal joint flexion
Dorsal interossei
Palmar interossei
Abductor digiti minimi

Flexor digit minimi
Flexor pollicis longus
Flexor pollicis brevis
Flexor digitorum profundus
Flexor digitorum superficialis
Adductor pollicis

Interphalangeal joint flexion
Flexor digitorum profundus
Flexor digitorum superficialis
Flexor pollicis longus

Metacarpophalangeal joint extension
Extensor digitorum communis
Extensor indicis
Extensor digiti minimi
Extensor pollicis longus
Extensor pollicis brevis

Interphalangeal joint extension
Lumbricals
Dorsal interossei
Palmar interossei
Extensor digiti minimi
Extensor digitorum communis
Extensor indicis
Extensor pollicis longus

Thumb carpometacarpal joint flexion
Flexor pollicis longus
Flexor pollicis brevis
Opponens pollicis

Thumb interphalangeal joint flexion
Flexor pollicis longus

Thumb carpometacarpal joint extension
Extensor pollicis longus
Abductor pollicis longus
Extensor pollicis brevis

Thumb interphalangeal joint extension
Extensor pollicis longus
Abductor pollicis brevis

Thumb carpometacarpal abduction
Abductor pollicis brevis
Abductor pollicis longus
Extensor pollicis brevis

Thumb carpometacarpal adduction
Adductor pollicis

Thumb carpometacarpal opposition
Opponens pollicis
Abductor pollicis brevis
Flexor pollicis brevis

23. BRACHIORADIALIS

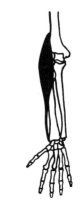

Origin
- Upper two-thirds of the lateral supracondylar ridge of the humerus
- Lateral intermuscular septum

Insertion
- Lateral surface of the radius just proximal to the base of the styloid process

Roots C5-6

Trunk Upper

Cord Posterior

Nerve Radial

Copyright © 1997, McGraw-Hill.

Open Chain Actions

SOLO ACTION
- Elbow flexion

COMBINED ACTION
- Supination to midposition
- Pronation to midposition

Closed Chain Action With the forearm fixed, brings the arm toward the forearm.

Synergists

Muscle	Nerve	Root
• Biceps brachii [20]	Musculocutaneous	C5-6
• Brachialis [21]	Musculocutaneous, radial	C5-7
• Supinator [24]	Radial (posterior interosseus)	C5-6
• Pronator teres [32]	Median	C6-7
• Pronator quadratus 38]	Median (anterior interosseus)	C7-T1
• Flexor carpi radialis [33]	Median	C6-8
• Flexor carpi ulnaris [50]	Ulnar	C8-T1
• Palmaris longus [34]	Median	C7-T1
• Flexor digitorum superficialis [35]	Median	C7-T1

Antagonists

Muscle	Nerve	Root
• Triceps brachii and anconeus [22]	Radial	C6-8
• Extensor carpi radialis longus and brevis [25]	Radial	C6-7
• Extensor carpi ulnaris [27]	Radial (posterior interosseus)	C6-8
• Extensor digitorum communis [26]	Radial (posterior interosseus)	C6-8

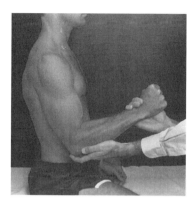

MUSCLE TESTING INSTRUCTIONS

Patient

Sitting or supine: With the forearm placed in a neutral position half way between supination and pronation, the patient flexes the elbow.

Tester

The tester is sitting or standing in front of the patient, placing one hand at the elbow to stabilize it.

Test

"Bend your elbow."

Pitfalls

The forearm must be kept in a neutral position; otherwise, the brachioradialis will not be isolated.

CLINICAL PEARLS

1. The brachioradialis [23] muscle is a very good C5-6, radial nerve innervated muscle. This anatomic fact makes the brachioradialis [23] useful in electrodiagnosis and manual muscle testing,

24. SUPINATOR

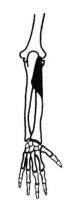

Origin
- Lateral epicondyle of the humerus
- Supinator crest of the ulna
- Radial collateral ligament of the elbow
- Annular ligament of the radial ulnar joint

Insertion
- Lateral aspect of the upper third of the radius, extensively covering the anterior and posterior surfaces

Roots C5-6

Trunk Upper

Cord Posterior

Nerve Radial

Open Chain Actions
SOLO ACTION
- Supination

COMBINED ACTION N/A

Closed Chain Action N/A

Synergists

Muscle	Nerve	Root
• Biceps brachii [20]	Musculocutaneous	C5-6
• Brachioradialis [23]	Radial	C5-6

Antagonists

Muscle	Nerve	Root
• Pronator teres [32]	Median	C6-7
• Pronator quadratus [38]	Median (anterior interosseus)	C7-T1
• Brachioradialis [23]	Radial	C5-6
• Flexor carpi radialis [33]	Median	C6-8

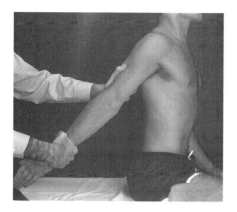

MUSCLE TESTING INSTRUCTIONS

Patient

Sitting, standing, or supine:

Technique 1: The patient completely flexes the elbow and flexes the shoulder to 90 degrees. The patient supinates the forearm.

Technique 2: The patient completely extends the elbow (in order to put the biceps brachii [20] at a mechanical disadvantage). The patient supinates the forearm.

Tester

The tester is either in front of or behind the patient.

Technique 1: With the elbow completely flexed, the shoulder is flexed to 90 degrees. One hand is placed on the extensor surface of the flexed elbow and the other hand on the distal forearm just proximal to the wrist.

Technique 2: With the fully extended position, one hand should be placed at the distal forearm just proximal to the wrist and the other hand on the extensor surface of the elbow.

Test

"Turn your forearm out against my hand."

Pitfalls

If the shoulder and elbow are not properly flexed (or extended), the biceps brachii [20] will contribute to supination and the supinator [24] will not have been isolated.

CLINICAL PEARLS

1. Supinator [24] weakness results in inability to hold the test position.
2. In "supinator syndrome," it is technically possible that the supinator [24] muscle will be normal in electrodiagnosis and manual muscle testing, as the radial nerve often sends branches to this muscle prior to diving into the arcade of Frohse.

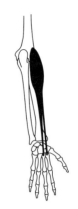

25. EXTENSOR CARPI RADIALIS LONGUS AND BREVIS (ECRL&B)

Origin
- Extensor carpi radialis longus: Lower third of the lateral supracondylar ridge of the humerus
- Extensor carpi radialis brevis: Lateral epicondlye of the humerus

Insertion
- Extensor carpi radialis longus: Dorsal surface of the base of the 2d metacarpal
- Extensor carpi radialis brevis: Dorsal surface of the base of the 3d metacarpal

Roots C6-7

Trunk Upper and middle

Cord Posterior

Nerve Radial

Open Chain Actions

SOLO ACTION
- Wrist extension
- Wrist radial deviation

COMBINED ACTION
- Elbow flexion (extensor carpi radialis longus)
- Finger flexion (indirectly, see below)

Closed Chain Action Stabilizes the wrist during activities such as the chin up.

Synergists

Muscle	Nerve	Root
• Extensor carpi ulnaris [27]	Posterior interosseus (radial)	C6-8
• Flexor carpi radialis [33]	Median	C6-8
• Extensor digitorum communis [26]	Posterior interosseus (radial)	C6-8
• Extensor indicis [28]	Posterior interosseus (radial)	C6-8
• Extensor pollicis longus [29]	Posterior interosseus (radial)	C6-8
• Extensor pollis brevis [31]	Posterior interosseus (radial)	C6-8
• Abductor pollicis longus [30]	Posterior interosseus (radial)	C6-8

Antagonists

Muscle	Nerve	Root
• Extensor carpi ulnaris [27]	Posterior interosseus (radial)	C6-8
• Flexor carpi ulnaris [50]	Ulnar	C8-T1
• Flexor carpi radialis [33]	Median	C6-8
• Palmaris longus [34]	Median	C7-T1
• Flexor digitorum profundus [37]	Anterior interosseus (median); ulnar	C7-T1
• Flexor digitorum superficialis [35]	Median	C7-T1
• Flexor pollicis longus [36]	Anterior interosseus (median)	C7-T1

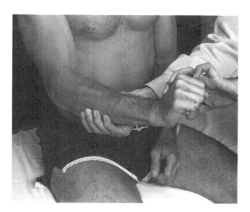

MUSCLE TESTING INSTRUCTIONS

Patient

The patient is sitting or supine with the forearm just short of full pronation. The forearm and wrist are supported by the examiner or the table. The patient extends the wrist in a radial direction.

Tester

The tester may be standing or sitting in front of the patient, applying pressure on the dorsum of the hand along the 2d metacarpal bone. The tester generates pressure so as to flex the wrist in an ulnar direction. Palpate at the base of the 2d metacarpal to test the extensor carpi radialis longus and palpate at the base of the 3d metacarpal to test the extensor carpi radialis brevis.

Test

"Pull your wrist up against my hand."

Pitfalls

N/A

CLINICAL PEARLS

1. The insertion of the extensor carpi radialis longus [25] into the base of the 2d metacarpal bone is easily palpated on the dorsum of the hand.
2. The insertion of the extensor carpi radialis brevis [25] into the base of the 3d metacarpal bone is easily palpated on the dorsum of the hand.
3. In a normal situation, the fingers will passively flex during wrist extension. If instead, the fingers extend, this might be a substitution maneuver for weak wrist extensors.
4. Wrist extension brings about passive finger flexion via a tenodesis action.

26. EXTENSOR DIGITORUM COMMUNIS

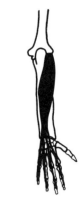

Origin
- Lateral epicondyle of the humerus

Insertion
- Four tendons of this muscle separate after crossing the wrist and in a variable fashion attach to the dorsum of digits 2 to 5.
  - The intermediate or middle slip inserts into the dorsal surface of the base of the middle phalanges.
  - The two lateral or collateral slips reunite over the middle phalanx and insert into the dorsum of the base of the distal phalanges.

Roots C6-8

Trunk Upper, middle, and lower

Cord Posterior

Nerve Posterior interosseus (radial)

Open Chain Actions
SOLO ACTION
- Extension of metacarpophalangeal joints 2 to 5
- Extension of interphalangeal joints 2 to 5

COMBINED ACTION
- Wrist extension
- Abduction of digits 2, 4, and 5 during wrist extension

Closed Chain Action N/A

Synergists

Muscle	Nerve	Root
• Extensor carpi radialis longus and brevis [25]	Radial	C6-7
• Extensor carpi ulnaris [27]	Posterior interosseus (radial)	C6-8
• Extensor indicis [28]	Posterior interosseus (radial)	C6-8
• Extensor pollicis longus [29]	Posterior interosseus (radial)	C6-8
• Lumbricals [42]	Median, ulnar	C7-T1
• Interossei [47,48]	Ulnar	C8-T1

Antagonists

Muscle	Nerve	Root
• Flexor carpi radialis [33]	Median	C6-8
• Flexor carpi ulnaris [50]	Ulnar	C8-T1
• Palmaris longus [34]	Median	C7-T1
• Flexor digitorum profundus [37]	Anterior interosseus (median), ulnar	C7-T1
• Flexor digitorum superficialis [35]	Median	C7-T1
• Flexor pollicis longus [36]	Anterior interosseus (median)	C7-T1
• Lumbricals [42]	Median, ulnar	C8, T1
• Interossei [47,48]	Ulnar	C8-T1
• Abductor digiti minimi [44]	Ulnar	C8-T1
• Flexor digiti minimi [45]	Ulnar	C8-T1
• Opponens digiti minimi [43]	Ulnar	C8-T1

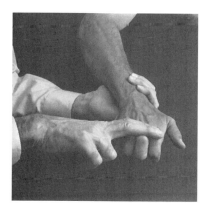

MUSCLE TESTING INSTRUCTIONS

Patient

Supine or sitting; the forearm is pronated with the wrist half way between flexion and extension (neutral position). The MCP and IP joints should be mildly flexed. The patient extends the MCPs.

Tester

The tester stabilizes the wrist with one hand and, with the other hand, generates pressure against the dorsal surfaces of the patient's proximal phalanges with one or two fingers.

Test

"Push your fingers up against mine."

Pitfalls

Lack of appropriate wrist stabilization allows for substitution by other muscles.

CLINICAL PEARLS

1. Contracture of the extensor digitorum communis [26] results in a hyperextension deformity of the metacarpophalangeal joints.

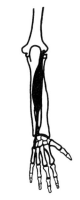

27. EXTENSOR CARPI ULNARIS

Origin
- Lateral epicondyle of the humerus
- Middle third of the narrow ridge on the dorsal border of the ulna

Insertion
- Posterior surface of the base of the 5th metacarpal

Roots C6-8

Trunk Upper, middle, and lower

Cord Posterior

Nerve Posterior interosseus (radial)

Open Chain Actions
SOLO ACTION
- Wrist extension
- Wrist ulnar deviation

COMBINED ACTION N/A

Closed Chain Action Stabilizes the wrist in activities such as a chin up

Synergists

Muscle	Nerve	Root
• Flexor carpi ulnaris [50]	Ulnar	C8-T1
• Flexor pollicis longus [36]	Anterior interosseus (median)	C8-T1
• Extensor carpi radialis longus and brevis [25]	Radial	C6-7
• Extensor digitorum communis [26]	Posterior interosseus (radial)	C6-8
• Extensor indicis [28]	Posterior interosseus (radial)	C6-8
• Extensor pollicis longus [29]	Posterior interosseus (radial)	C6-8

Antagonists

Muscle	Nerve	Root
• Flexor carpi radialis [33]	Median	C6-8
• Extensor carpi radialis longus and brevis [25]	Radial	C6-7
• Extensor pollicis brevis [31]	Posterior interosseus (radial)	C6-8
• Abductor pollicis longus [30]	Posterior interosseus (radial)	C6-8
• Flexor carpi ulnaris [50]	Ulnar	C8-T1
• Palmaris longus [34]	Median	C7-T1
• Flexor digitorum profundus [37]	Anterior interosseus (median), ulnar	C7-T1
• Flexor digitorum superficialis [35]	Median	C7-T1
• Flexor pollicis longus [36]	Median	C7-T1

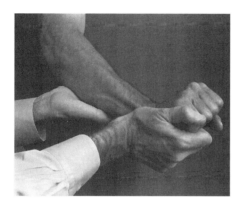

MUSCLE TESTING INSTRUCTIONS

Patient
Sitting or supine with forearm completely pronated, the patient extends the wrist in an ulnar direction.

Tester
The tester is in front of or to the side of the patient. With one hand, the tester supports the patient's forearm and with the other hand generates pressure to the dorsum of the hand along the patient's 5th metacarpal bone. Such pressure should be directed in a radial vector.

Test
"Bring your hand up and out against my hand."

Pitfalls
N/A

CLINICAL PEARLS

1. In a normal situation, the fingers will passively flex during wrist extension. If instead, the fingers extend, this might be a substitution maneuver for weak wrist extensors.
2. Wrist extension brings about passive finger flexion via a tenodesis action.

28. EXTENSOR INDICIS

Origin
- Dorsal surface of the lower half of the body of the ulna
- Interosseus membrane

Insertion
- Ulnar side of the tendon of the index finger of the extensor digitorum communis [26] and into the dorsal expansion of the finger extensor tendons

Roots C6-C8

Trunk Upper, middle, and lower

Cord Posterior

Nerve Posterior interosseus (radial)

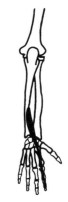

Copyright © 1997, McGraw-Hill.

Open Chain Actions
SOLO ACTION
- Extension of metacarpophalangeal joint of 2d digit
- Extension of interphalangeal joints of 2d digit

COMBINED ACTION
- Wrist extension
- Abduction of metacarpophalangeal joint of 2d digit

Closed Chain Action N/A

Synergists

Muscle	Nerve	Root
• Extensor carpi radialis longus and brevis [25]	Radial	C6-7
• Extensor carpi ulnaris [27]	Posterior interosseus (radial)	C6-8
• Extensor digitorum communis [26]	Posterior interosseus (radial)	C6-8
• Extensor pollicis longus [29]	Posterior interosseus (radial)	C6-8
• Lumbricals [42]	Median, ulnar	C7-T1
• Interossei [47,48]	Ulnar	C8-T1

Antagonists

Muscle	Nerve	Root
• Flexor carpi radialis [33]	Median	C6-8
• Flexor carpi ulnaris [50]	Ulnar	C8-T1
• Palmaris longus [34]	Median	C7-T1
• Flexor digitorum profundus [37]	Anterior interosseus (median), ulnar	C7-T1
• Flexor digitorum superficialis [35]	Median	C7-T1
• Flexor pollicis longus [36]	Anterior interosseus (median)	C7-T1
• Lumbricals [42]	Median, ulnar	C7-T1
• Interossei [47,48]	Ulnar	C8-T1

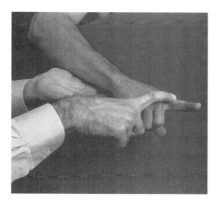

MUSCLE TESTING INSTRUCTIONS

Patient

Sitting or supine, the patient extends the index finger.

Tester

The tester is in front or to the side of the patient and stabilizes the wrist of the patient. Pressure is generated in a flexion vector to the dorsum of the proximal phalanx of the index finger.

Test

"Raise your index finger up."

Pitfalls

N/A

CLINICAL PEARLS

1. The extensor indicis [28] is the distalmost muscle innervated by the radial nerve.

29. EXTENSOR POLLICIS LONGUS

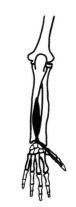

Origin
- Posterior surface of the middle third of the ulna
- Interosseus membrane

Insertion
- Posterior surface of the base of the distal phalanx of the thumb

Roots C6-C8

Trunk Upper, middle, and lower

Cord Posterior

Nerve Posterior interosseus (radial)

Open Chain Actions
SOLO ACTION
- Extension of metacarpophalangeal joint of 1st digit (thumb)
- Extension of interpalangeal joint of 1st digit (thumb)
- Extension of carpometacarpal of 1st digit (thumb)

COMBINED ACTION
- Wrist radial deviation
- Wrist abduction
- Wrist extension

Closed Chain Action N/A

Synergists

Muscle	Nerve	Root
• Abductor pollicis brevis [39]	Median	C7-T1
• Flexor pollicis brevis [41]	Median, ulnar	C7-T1
• Adductor pollicis [46]	Ulnar	C8-T1
• 1st Palmar interosseus [47]	Ulnar	C8-T1
• Extensor carpi radialis longus and brevis [25]	Radial	C6-7
• Extensor carpi ulnaris [27]	Posterior interosseus (radial)	C6-8
• Extensor digitorum communis [26]	Radial	C6-8
• Extensor indicis [28]	Radial	C6-8

Antagonists

Muscle	Nerve	Root
• Flexor pollicis longus [36]	Anterior interosseus (median)	C7-T1
• Flexor pollicis brevis [41]	Median, Ulnar	C7-T1
• Abductor pollicis brevis [39]	Median	C7-T1
• Flexor carpi radialis [33]	Median	C6-8
• Flexor carpi ulnaris [50]	Ulnar	C8-T1
• Palmaris longus [34]	Median	C7-T1
• Flexor digitorum profundus [37]	Anterior interosseus (median), ulnar	C7-T1
• Flexor digitorum superficialis [35]	Median	C7-T1

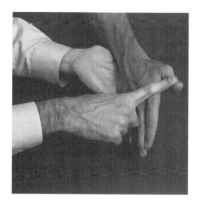

MUSCLE TESTING INSTRUCTIONS

Patient

Sitting or supine, the patient extends the thumb.

Tester

The tester is in front of or to the side of the patient. The patient's hand is stabilized by the tester. The tester's index finger generates a flexion vector to the distal phalanx of the dorsal surface of the thumb.

Test

"Push your thumb back against my finger."

Pitfalls

N/A

CLINICAL PEARLS

1. By virtue of the attachment of the abductor pollicis brevis [30], flexor pollicis brevis [41], adductor pollicis [46], and first palmar interosseus [46] into the extensor expansion of the thumb, theses muscles can extend the interphalangeal joint of the thumb.

30. ABDUCTOR POLLICIS LONGUS

Origin
- Posterior surface of the distal two-thirds of the ulna
- Posterior surface of the middle third of the radius
- Interosseus membrane

Insertion
- Radial side of the base of the first metacarpal

Roots C6-C8

Trunk Upper, middle, and lower

Cord Posterior

Nerve Posterior interosseus (radial)

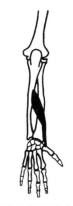

Copyright © 1997, McGraw-Hill.

Open Chain Actions
SOLO ACTION
- Abduction of the carpometacarpal joint of the thumb
- Extension of the carpometacarpal joint of the thumb

COMBINED ACTION
- Wrist radial deviation
- Wrist flexion

Closed Chain Action N/A

Synergists

Muscle	Nerve	Root
• Flexor carpi radialis [33]	Median	C6-8
• Extensor carpi radialis longus and brevis [25]	Radial	C6-7
• Abductor pollicis brevis [39]	Medial	C7-T1
• Extensor pollicis brevis [31]	Posterior interosseus (radial)	C6-8

Antagonists

Muscle	Nerve	Root
• Flexor carpi ulnaris [50]	Ulnar	C8-T1
• Extensor carpi ulnaris [27]	Posterior interosseus (radial)	C6-8
• Flexor pollicis longus [36]	Anterior interosseus (median)	C7-T1
• Flexor pollicis brevis [41]	Median, ulnar	C7-T1
• Adductor pollicis [46]	Ulnar	C8-T1

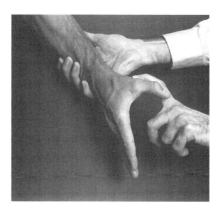

MUSCLE TESTING INSTRUCTIONS

Patient

Sitting or supine, the patient abducts the thumb.

Tester

The tester is in front of or to the side of the patient while stabilizing the patient's wrist. The 1st metacarpal bone in placed in abduction and slight extension. Pressure is generated in an adduction and flexion vector against the lateral aspect of the distal 1st metacarpal.

Test

"Push your thumb out against my finger."

Pitfalls

N/A

CLINICAL PEARLS

1. This muscle forms one of the boundaries of the "anatomic snuff box."

31. EXTENSOR POLLICIS BREVIS

Origin
- Dorsal surface of the distal third of the radius
- Interosseus membrane

Insertion
- Dorsal surface of the base of the proximal phalanx of the thumb

Roots C6-8

Trunk Upper, middle, and lower

Cord Posterior

Nerve Posterior interosseus (radial)

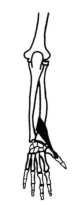

Copyright © 1997, McGraw-Hill.

Open Chain Actions
SOLO ACTION
- Extension of the metacarpophalangeal joint of the thumb
- Abduction of the carpometacarpal joint of the thumb
- Extension of carpometacarpal joint of the thumb

COMBINED ACTION
- Wrist radial deviation

Closed Chain Action N/A

Synergists

Muscle	Nerve	Root
• Flexor carpi radialis [33]	Median	C6-8
• Extensor carpi radialis longus and brevis [25]	Radial	C6-7
• Abductor pollicis longus [30]	Posterior interosseus (radial)	C6-8
• Abductor pollicis brevis [39]	Median	C7-T1

Antagonists

Muscle	Nerve	Root
• Flexor carpi ulnaris [50]	Ulnar	C8-T1
• Extensor carpi ulnaris [27]	Posterior interosseus (radial)	C6-8
• Flexor pollicis longus [36]	Anterior interosseus (median)	C7-T1
• Flexor pollicis brevis [41]	Median, ulnar	C7-T1
• Adductor pollicis [46]	Ulnar	C8-T1

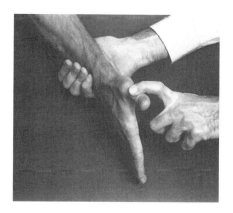

MUSCLE TESTING INSTRUCTIONS

Patient
Sitting or supine, the metacarpophalangeal joint of the thumb is extended.

Tester
The tester is in front of or to the side of the patient, stabilizing the wrist of the patient. The tester generates pressure in a flexion vector against the proximal phalanx.

Test
"Push out against my finger."

Pitfalls
N/A

CLINICAL PEARLS

1. This muscle tendon forms one of the boundaries of the "anatomic snuff box."

32. PRONATOR TERES

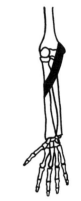

Origin
- One head from the medial epicondyle of the humerus
- The other head from the coronoid process of the ulna

Insertion
- Lateral surface of the radius near its center

Roots C6-7

Trunk Upper and middle

Cord Lateral and medial

Nerve Median

Open Chain Actions
SOLO ACTION
- Pronates the forearm

COMBINED ACTION
- Elbow flexion

Closed Chain Action Assists in approximating the arm and the forearm during a chin-up

Synergists

Muscle	Nerve	Root
• Biceps brachii [20]	Musculocutaneous	C5-6
• Brachialis [21]	Musculocutaneous, radial	C5-7
• Brachioradialis [23]	Radial	C5-6
• Flexor carpi radialis [33]	Median	C6-8
• Flexor carpi ulnaris [50]	Ulnar	C8-T1
• Palmaris longus [34]	Median	C7-T1
• Flexor digitorum superficialis [35]	Median	C7-T1
• Pronator quadratus [38]	Anterior interosseus (median)	C7-T1

Antagonists

Muscle	Nerve	Root
• Triceps brachii and anconeus [22]	Radial	C6-8
• Biceps brachii [20]	Musculocutaneous	C5-6
• Brachioradialis [23]	Radial	C5-6
• Supinator [24]	Posterior interosseus (radial)	C5-6

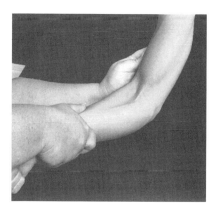

MUSCLE TESTING INSTRUCTIONS

Patient

Sitting or supine, with the elbow flexed to approximately 60 degrees; the forearm is pronated.

Tester

The tester is in front of or to the side of the patient, stabilizing the elbow against the patient's thorax in order to prevent any shoulder movement. The tester generates a supination vector distally on the forearm proximal to the wrist.

Test

"Turn your forearm in towards your body."

Pitfalls

If the elbow is flexed too much or too little, the pronator teres [32] is put at a mechanical disadvantage and will not be properly isolated.

CLINICAL PEARLS

1. It is important in this test to differentiate the functions of the pronator teres [32] from the pronator quadratus [38]; therefore, the elbow should be partially flexed and pressure generated proximal to the wrist.

33. FLEXOR CARPI RADIALIS

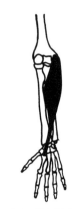

Origin
- Common flexor tendon from the medial epicondyle of the humerus
- Antebrachial fascia

Insertion
- Anterior surface of the base of the 2d metacarpal with a slip to the base of the 3d metacarpal

Roots C6-8

Trunk Upper, middle, and lower

Cord Lateral and medial

Nerve Median

Open Chain Actions
SOLO ACTION
- Wrist flexion
- Wrist radial deviation

COMBINED ACTION
- Elbow flexion
- Possible weak forearm pronation

Closed Chain Action Contributes to approximating the arm to the forearm during a chin-up

Synergists

Muscle	Nerve	Root
• Flexor carpi ulnaris [50]	Ulnar	C8-T1
• Palmaris longus [34]	Median	C7-T1
• Flexor digitorum profundus [37]	Anterior interosseus (median), ulnar	C7-T1
• Flexor digitorum superficialis [35]	Median	C7-T1
• Flexor pollicis longus [36]	Anterior interosseus (median)	C7-T1
• Extensor carpi radialis longus and brevis [25]	Radial	C6-7
• Extensor pollicis brevis [31]	Posterior interosseus (radial)	C6-8
• Abductor pollicis longus [30]	Posterior interosseus (radial)	C6-8

Antagonists

Muscle	Nerve	Root
• Flexor carpi ulnaris [50]	Ulnar	C8-T1
• Extensor carpi ulnaris [27]	Posterior interosseus (radial)	C6-8
• Flexor pollicis longus [36]	Anterior interosseus (median)	C7-T1
• Extensor carpi radialis longus and brevis [25]	Radial	C6-7
• Extensor digitorum communis [26]	Posterior interosseus (radial)	C6-8
• Extensor indicis [28]	Posterior interosseus (radial)	C6-8
• Extensor pollicis longus [29]	Posterior interosseus (radial)	C6-8

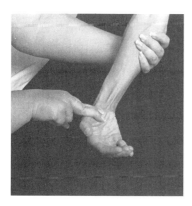

MUSCLE TESTING INSTRUCTIONS

Patient
Sitting or supine, the patient flexes and ulnarly deviates the wrist while the forearm is in supination.

Tester
The tester is positioned in front of or to the side of the patient, holding the forearm of the patient near full supination. The tester generates an ulnar and extension vector against the thenar eminence.

Test
"Push your hand up against my hand."

Pitfalls
N/A

CLINICAL PEARLS

1. At the wrist, the median nerve is found between the tendon of this muscle and that of the palmaris longus [34].

34. PALMARIS LONGUS

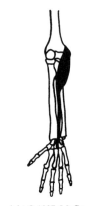

Origin
- Common flexor tendon from the medial epicondyle of the humerus
- Antebrachial fascia

Insertion
- Palmar aponeurosis
- Flexor retinaculum of the wrist

Roots C7-T1

Trunk Middle and lower

Cord Lateral and medial

Nerve Median

Open Chain Actions
Solo Action
- Tenses the palmar fascia
- Wrist flexion

Combined Action
- Elbow flexion

Closed Chain Action N/A

Synergists

Muscle	Nerve	Root
• Flexor carpi radialis [33]	Median	C6-8
• Flexor carpi ulnaris [50]	Ulnar	C8-T1
• Flexor digitorum profundus [37]	Anterior interosseus (median), ulnar	C7-T1
• Flexor digitorum superficialis [35]	Median	C7-T1
• Flexor pollicis longus [36]	Anterior interosseus (median)	C7-T1

Antagonists

Muscle	Nerve	Root
• Extensor carpi ulnaris [27]	Posterior interosseus (radial)	C6-8
• Extensor carpi radialis longus and brevis [25]	Radial	C6-7
• Extensor digitorum communis [26]	Posterior interosseus (radial)	C6-8
• Extensor indicis [28]	Posterior Interosseus (radial)	C6-8
• Extensor pollicis longus [29]	Posterior interosseus (radial)	C6-8

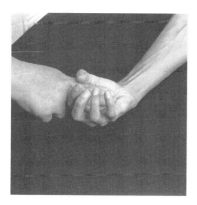

MUSCLE TESTING INSTRUCTIONS

Patient

Sitting or supine, the patient flexes the wrist and cups the palm.

Tester

The tester is in front of or to the side of the patient, with the patient's forearm resting on a table for support in a position of supination. The tester generates an extension vector to the wrist.

Test

"Cup your palm and push your hand up against me."

Pitfalls

N/A

CLINICAL PEARLS

1. A minority of the population does not have a palmaris longus [34] muscle.

35. FLEXOR DIGITORUM SUPERFICIALIS

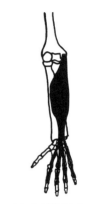

Origin
- Common flexor tendon from the medial epicondyle of the humerus
- Coronoid process of the ulna
- Along oblique line on the middle half of the anterior surface of the radius

Insertion
- Four tendons that separate after passing the wrist. Each tendon separates into two parts that insert into the sides of the base of the middle phalanges of digits 2 to 5.

Copyright © 1997, McGraw-Hill.

Roots C7-T1

Trunk Middle and lower

Cord Lateral and medial

Nerve Median

Open Chain Actions

SOLO ACTION
- Metacarpophalangeal flexion digits 2 to 5
- Interphalangeal flexion of the proximal interphalengeal (PIP) joint for digits 2 to 5

COMBINED ACTION
- Wrist flexion

Closed Chain Action N/A

Synergists

Muscle	Nerve	Root
• Flexor digitorum profundus [37]	Anterior interosseus (median), ulnar	C7-T1
• Flexor carpi radialis [33]	Median	C6-8
• Flexor carpi ulnaris [50]	Ulnar	C8-T1
• Palmaris longus [34]	Median	C7-T1
• Lumbricals [42]	Median, ulnar	C7-T1
• Interossei [47,48]	Ulnar	C8-T1
• Abductor digiti minimi [44]	Ulnar	C8-T1
• Flexor digiti minimi [45]	Ulnar	C8-T1
• Opponens digiti minimi [43]	Ulnar	C8-T1

Antagonists

Muscle	Nerve	Root
• Extensor carpi radialis longus and brevis [25]	Radial	C6-7
• Extensor carpi ulnaris [27]	Posterior interosseus (radial)	C6-8
• Extensor digitorum communis [26]	Posterior interosseus (radial)	C6-8
• Extensor indicis [28]	Posterior interosseus (radial)	C6-8
• Lumbricals [42]	Median, ulnar	C7-T1
• Interossei [47,48]	Ulnar	C8-T1

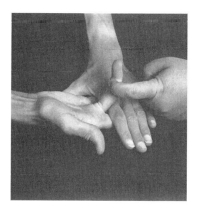

MUSCLE TESTING INSTRUCTIONS

Patient
Sitting or supine, the patient bends the middle phalanx of the finger.

Tester
The tester is in front of or to the side of the patient. With the patient's forearm resting on a supporting surface in supination, the metacarpophalangeal joint is stabilized. The wrist should not be allowed to flex. With each finger tested individually, the tester generates an extension vector to the volar aspect of the middle phalanx.

Test
"Curl your finger in against mine."

Pitfalls
N/A

CLINICAL PEARLS

1. The flexor digitorum superficialis [35] is best isolated if the three fingers that are not being tested are put into maximum extension. In this manner the flexor digitorum profundus [37] is placed at a mechanical disadvantage.

36. FLEXOR POLLICIS LONGUS

Origin
- Anterior surface of the middle half of the radius
- Adjacent parts of the interosseus membrane
- Coronoid process of ulna
- Possibly the medial epicondyle of the humerus

Insertion
- Palmar surface of the base of the distal phalanx of the thumb

Roots C7-T1

Trunk Middle and lower

Cord Lateral and medial

Nerve Anterior interosseus (median)

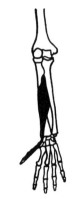

Open Chain Actions
SOLO ACTION
- Flexion of interphalangeal joint of the thumb

COMBINED ACTION
- Flexion of the metacarpophlangeal joint of the thumb
- Flexion of the carpometacarpophalangeal joint of the thumb
- Wrist flexion

Closed Chain Action N/A

Synergists

Muscle	Nerve	Root
• Flexor carpi radialis [33]	Median	C6-8
• Flexor carpi ulnaris [50]	Ulnar	C8-T1
• Palmaris longus [34]	Median	C7-T1
• Flexor digitorum profundus [37]	Anterior interosseus (median), ulnar	C7-T1
• Flexor digitorum superficialis [35]	Median	C7-T1
• Flexor pollicis brevis [41]	Median, ulnar	C7-T1
• Abductor pollicis brevis [39]	Median	C7-T1
• Adductor pollicis [46]	Ulnar	C8-T1

Antagonists

Muscle	Nerve	Root
• Extensor carpi radialis longus and brevis [25]	Radial	C6-7
• Extensor carpi ulnaris [27]	Posterior interosseus (radial)	C6-8
• Extensor digitorum communis [26]	Posterior interosseus (radial)	C6-8
• Extensor indicis [28]	Posterior interosseus (radial)	C6-8
• Extensor pollicis longus [29]	Posterior interosseus (radial)	C6-8
• Extensor pollicis brevis [31]	Posterior interosseus (radial)	C6-8
• Abductor pollicis brevis [39]	Median	C7-T1
• Abductor pollicis longus [30]	Posterior interosseus (radial)	C6-8

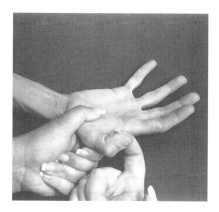

MUSCLE TESTING INSTRUCTIONS

Patient
Sitting or supine, the hand is resting on a surface in forearm supination. The patient bends the distal phalanx of the thumb.

Tester
The tester is in front of or to the side of the patient and stabilizes the metacarpophalangeal joint of the thumb in extension. With the other hand, the tester generates an extension vector to the volar aspect of the distal phalanx.

Test
"Push against my finger."

Pitfalls
N/A

CLINICAL PEARLS

1. Weakness of the flexor pollicis longus [36] makes it difficult to hold a pencil for writing or to pick up small objects between the thumb and fingers.
2. The flexor pollicis longus [36] is involved in the anterior interosseus syndrome.
3. Rupture of the tendon of the flexor pollicis longus [36] should be differentiated from weakness as would be seen in anterior interosseus syndrome.

37. FLEXOR DIGITORUM PROFUNDUS

Origin
- Anterior and medial surfaces of the proximal ulna
- Antebrachial fascia and interosseus membrane

Insertion
- Four tendons that separate after passing the wrist and go to digits 2 to 5. Each tendon passes through the split in the corresponding flexor digitorum superficialis tendon and is inserted into the volar surface of the base of the distal palanx

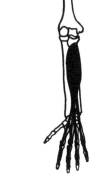

Roots C7-T1

Trunk Middle and lower

Cord Lateral and medial

Nerve
- Anterior interosseus (median) (digits 2 to 3)
- Ulnar (digits 4 to 5)

Open Chain Actions
SOLO ACTION
- Distal interphalangeal joint flexion digits 2 to 5

COMBINED ACTION
- Proximal interphalangeal joint flexion digits 2 to 5
- Adducts fingers toward midline
- Metacarpophalangeal flexion
- Wrist flexion

Closed Chain Action N/A

Synergists

Muscle	Nerve	Root
• Flexor carpi radialis [33]	Median	C6-8
• Flexor carpi ulnaris [50]	Ulnar	C8-T1
• Palmaris longus [34]	Median	C7-T1
• Flexor digitorum superficiais [35]	Median	C7-T1
• Flexor pollicis longus [36]	Anterior interosseus (median)	C7-T1
• Lumbricals [42]	Median, ulnar	C7-T1
• Interossei [47,48]	Ulnar	C8-T1
• Abductor digiti minimi [44]	Ulnar	C8-T1
• Flexor digiti minimi [45]	Ulnar	C8-T1
• Opponens digiti minimi [43]	Ulnar	C8-T1

Antagonists

Muscle	Nerve	Root
• Extensor carpi radialis longus and brevis [25]	Radial	C6-7
• Extensor carpi unlaris [27]	Posterior interosseus (radial)	C6-8
• Extensor digitorum communis [26]	Posterior interosseus (radial)	C6-8
• Extensor indicis [28]	Posterior interosseus (radial)	C6-8
• Extensor pollicis longus [29]	Posterior interosseus (radial)	C6-8
• Lumbricals [42]	Median, ulnar	C7-T1
• Interossei [47,48]	Ulnar	C8-T1

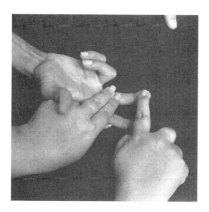

MUSCLE TESTING INSTRUCTIONS

Patient
Sitting or supine with the wrist in a neutral position or slightly extended, the patient flexes the distal phalanx.

Tester
The tester is in front of or to the side of the patient, stabilizing the middle and proximal phalanges. The tester generates an extension vector to the volar aspect of the distal phalanx. Each finger should be tested individually.

Test
"Push the tip of your finger against mine."

Pitfalls
N/A

CLINICAL PEARLS

1. The flexor digitorum profundus [37] of digits 2 and 3 is involved in the anterior interosseus syndrome.

38. PRONATOR QUADRATUS

Origin
- Distal fourth of the anterior surface of the ulna

Insertion
- Distal fourth of the anterior surface of the radius

Roots C7-T1

Trunk Middle and lower

Cord Lateral and medial

Nerve Anterior interosseus (median)

Open Chain Actions
SOLO ACTION
- Forearm pronation
COMBINED ACTION N/A

Closed Chain Action N/A

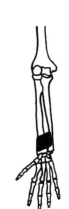

Copyright © 1997, McGraw-Hill.

Synergists

Muscle	Nerve	Root
• Pronator teres [32]	Median	C6-7
• Brachioradialis [23]	Radial	C5-6
• Flexor carpi radialis [33]	Median	C6-8

Antagonists

Muscle	Nerve	Root
• Biceps brachii [20]	Musculocutaneous	C5-6
• Brachioradialis [23]	Radial	C5-6
• Supinator [24]	Radial	C5-6

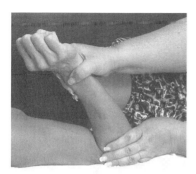

MUSCLE TESTING INSTRUCTIONS

Patient
Sitting or supine with the elbow completely flexed, the patient pronates the forearm.

Tester
The tester is in front of or to the side of the patient and stabilizes the arm by holding the elbow against the patient's thorax in order to deter shoulder movements. While the distal forearm is securely grasped, the tester generates a supination vector to the forearm.

Test
"Turn your forearm out."

Pitfalls
If the elbow is not held securely to the side, it is more likely that shoulder substitutions will occur.

CLINICAL PEARLS

1. This muscle is involved in the anterior interosseus syndrome.
2. This is the distalmost muscle innervated by the median nerve proximal to the carpal tunnel.

39. ABDUCTOR POLLICIS BREVIS

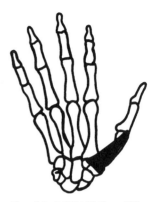

Origin
- Tuberosity of the scaphoid
- Ridge of the trapezium
- A slip from the transverse carpal ligament

Insertion
- Lateral surface of the base of the proximal phalanx of the thumb

Roots C7-T1

Trunk Middle and lower

Cord Lateral and medial

Nerve Median

Open Chain Actions

SOLO ACTION
- Abduction of the metacarpophalangeal joint of the thumb
- Abduction of the carpometacarpal joint of the thumb

COMBINED ACTION
- Opposition of the metacarpophalangeal joint of the thumb
- Flexion of the metacarpophalangeal joint of the thumb
- Extension of the interphalangeal joint of the thumb by its insertion into the extensor hood

Closed Chain Action N/A

Synergists

Muscle	Nerve	Root
• Abductor pollicis longus [30]	Posterior interosseus (radial)	C6-8
• Flexor pollicis longus[36]	Anterior interosseus (radial)	C7-T1
• Flexor pollicis brevis [41]	Median, ulnar	C7-T1

Antagonists

Muscle	Nerve	Root
• Adductor pollicis [46]	Ulnar	C8-T1
• Extensor pollicis longus [29]	Posterior interosseus (radial)	C6-8

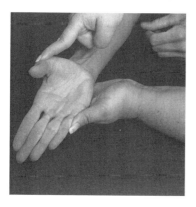

MUSCLE TESTING INSTRUCTIONS

Patient

Sitting or supine, the patient abducts the thumb.

Tester

The tester is in front of or to the side of the patient. The tester stabilizes the patient's hand and generates downward pressure against the proximal phalanx.

Test

"Push straight up against my finger."

Pitfalls

In order to properly isolate the abductor pollicis brevis [39], pressure must be applied over the proximal and not the distal phalanx.

CLINICAL PEARLS

1. Weakness of this muscle makes it difficult to grasp large objects.

40. OPPONENS POLLICIS

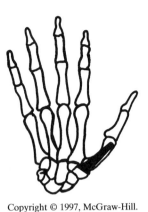

Origin
- Trapezium
- Transverse carpal ligament

Insertion
- Shaft of the 1st metacarpal on its radial side

Roots C7-T1

Trunk Middle and lower

Cord Lateral and medial

Nerve Median

Open Chain Actions

SOLO ACTION
- Opposition of carpometacarpal joint of the thumb

COMBINED ACTION N/A

Closed Chain Action N/A

Synergists

Muscle	Nerve	Root
• Flexor pollicis brevis [41]	Median, ulnar	C7-T1
• Adductor pollicis [46]	Ulnar	C8-T1

Antagonists

Muscle	Nerve	Root
• Extensor pollicis longus [29]	Posterior interosseus (radial)	C6-8
• Extensor pollicis brevis [31]	Posterior interosseus (radial)	C6-8

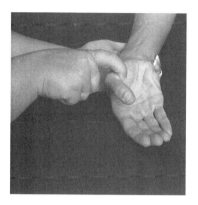

MUSCLE TESTING INSTRUCTIONS

Patient
Sitting or supine, the patient tries to touch his or her thumb to the little finger.

Tester
In front of or to the side of the patient, the tester stabilizes the patient's hand and generates pressure in an adduction and extension vector.

Test
"Bring the tip of your thumb to the base of your little finger."

Pitfalls
An examiner needs to know the definitions of the basic anatomical planes to carry out and understand this test.

CLINICAL PEARLS

1. Weakness of this muscle makes it difficult to grasp and hold objects between the thumb and fingers.

41. FLEXOR POLLICIS BREVIS (DEEP AND SUPERFICIAL HEADS)

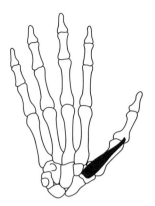

Origin
- Superficial head: Crest of the trapezium
- Deep head: Trapezoid and capitate bones and palmar ligaments of the distal row of the carpal bones

Insertion
- Base of the proximal phalanx of the thumb on the radial side and the extensor expansion

Roots C7-T1

Trunk Middle and lower

Cord Lateral and medial

Nerve
- Superficial head: Median
- Deep head: Ulnar

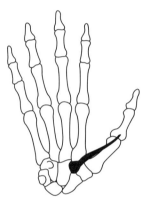

Open Chain Actions
SOLO ACTION
- Flexion of metacarpophalangeal flexion of digit 1
- Flexion of carpometacarpal of digit 1

COMBINED ACTION
- Assists in opposition of the thumb

Closed Chain Action N/A

Synergists

Muscle	Nerve	Root
• Flexor pollicis longus [36]	Anterior interosseus (median)	C8-T1
• Abductor pollicis brevis [39]	Median	C7-T1
• Adductor pollicis [46]	Ulnar	C8-T1

Antagonists

Muscle	Nerve	Root
• Extensor pollicis longus [29]	Posterior interosseus (radial)	C6-8
• Extensor pollicis brevis [31]	Posterior interosseus (radial)	C6-8

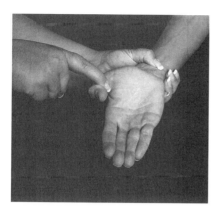

MUSCLE TESTING INSTRUCTIONS

Patient

Sitting or supine, the patient flexes the thumb.

Tester

In front of or to the side of the patient, the tester stabilizes the patient's hand and generates an extension vector to the volar surface of the proximal phalanx of the thumb.

Test

"Push your thumb in against my finger."

Pitfalls

An examiner needs to know the definitions of the basic anatomical planes to carry out and understand this test.

CLINICAL PEARLS

1. Weakness of this muscle makes it difficult to grasp and hold objects between the thumb and fingers.
2. With very marked weakness, a hyperextension deformity of the metacarpophalangeal joint is noted.
3. The flexor pollicis brevis [41] is a dually innervated muscle.

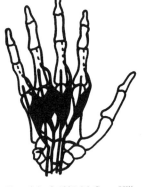

42. LUMBRICALS

Origin
- Tendons of the flexor digitorum profundus [37]

Insertion
- Extensor expansion on the dorsum of each digit along the radial side

Roots C7-T1

Trunk Middle and lower

Cord Lateral and medial

Nerve
- Lumbricals 1 and 2: 3d and 4th digital branches of the median nerve
- Lumbricals 3 and 4: Branches of the palmar branch of the ulnar nerve

Open Chain Actions
SOLO ACTION
- Flexion of the metacarpophalangeal joint of digits 2 to 5
- Extension of the distal and proximal interphalangeal joints of digits 2 to 5

COMBINED ACTION
- Abduction of the metacarpophalangeal joints of digits 2 to 5

Closed Chain Action N/A

Synergists

Muscle	Nerve	Root
• Dorsal interossei [48]	Ulnar	C8-T1
• Flexor digitorum profundus [37]	Ulnar, Anterior interosseus (median)	C7T1
• Flexor digitorum superficialis [35]	Median	C7-T1
• Abductor digiti minimi [44]	Ulnar	C8-T1
• Flexor digiti minimi [45]	Ulnar	C8-T1
• Opponens digiti minimi [43]	Ulnar	C8-T1
• Extensor digitorum communis [26]	Posterior interosseus (radial)	C6-8
• Extensor indicis [28]	Posterior interosseus (radial)	C6-8
• Palmar interossei [47]	Ulnar	C8-T1

Antagonists

Muscle	Nerve	Root
• Extensor digitorum communis [26]	Posterior interosseus (radial)	C6-8
• Extensor indicis [28]	Posterior interosseus (radial)	C6-8
• Palmar interossei [47]	Ulnar	C8-T1
• Flexor digitorum profundus [37]	Anterior interosseus (median), ulnar	C7-T1
• Flexor digitorum superficialis [35]	Median	C7-T1

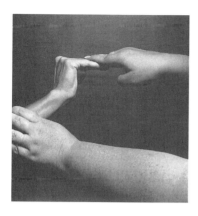 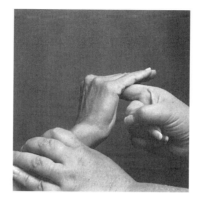

MUSCLE TESTING INSTRUCTIONS

Patient
Sitting or supine, the patient puts the hand into an intrinsic plus position.

Tester
The tester is in front of or to the side of the patient. With the wrist held securely in minimal extension, pressure is generated in two distinct phases. In the first phase, a flexion vector is generated to the dorsal surfaces of the distal and middle phalanges. Next, an extension vector is generated to the volar surfaces of the proximal phalanges.

Test
"Push your fingers against my finger."

Pitfalls
N/A

CLINICAL PEARLS

1. Weakness of the lumbricals [42] may result in a "Claw hand" deformity.

43. OPPONENS DIGITI MINIMI

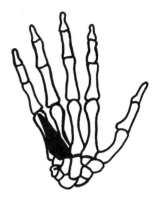

Origin
- Convex surface of the hamate bone
- Contiguous portion of the transverse carpal ligament

Insertion
- Ulnar aspect of the entire length of the metacarpal bone of the 5th digit

Roots C8-T1

Trunk Lower

Cord Medial

Nerve Ulnar

Open Chain Actions
SOLO ACTION
- Flexion of metacarpophalangeal joint of digit 5
- Rotation of the 5th metacarpal in "cupping" the hand

COMBINED ACTION N/A

Closed Chain Action N/A

Synergists

Muscle	Nerve	Root
• Flexor digiti minimi [45]	Ulnar	C8-T1
• Abductor digiti minimi [44]	Ulnar	C8-T1
• Lumbricals, 4th [42]	Ulnar	C7-T1
• Palmar interossei 3 to 4 [47]	Ulnar	C8-T1
• Flexor digitorum superficialis [35]	Median	C7-T1
• Flexor digitorum profundus [37]	Median, ulnar	C7-T1

Antagonists

Muscle	Nerve	Root
• Extensor digitorum communis [26]	Posterior intereosseus (radial)	C6-8
• Extensor digiti minimi	Posterior intereosseus (radial)	C6-8
• Abductor digiti minimi [44]	Ulnar	C8-T1

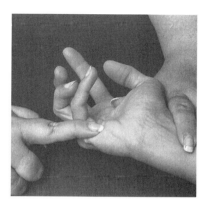

MUSCLE TESTING INSTRUCTIONS

Patient

Sitting or supine, the patient tries to cup the 5th metacarpal towards the thumb.

Tester

The tester is in front of or to the side of the patient. Grasping the hand firmly, the tester secures the 1st metacarpal bone. With the hand cupped, a downward pressure is generated to the 5th metacarpal.

Test

"Try to bring your little finger up and in to your thumb."

Pitfalls

N/A

CLINICAL PEARLS

1. Weakness of this muscle may result in a flattened appearance of the palm.
2. Although individual muscle antagonists were listed, these muscles must work in a group to provide a counterforce to the opponens digiti minimi [43].

44. ABDUCTOR DIGITI MINIMI

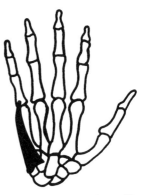

Origin
- Pisiform bone
- Tendon of the flexor carpi ulnaris [50]

Insertion This muscle inserts by two slips. Connections from each slip go to the dorsal expansion of the finger extensor tendons.
- One inserts into the ulnar side of the base of the proximal phalanx of the 5th digit.
- The other inserts into the ulnar border of the aponeurosis of the extensor digiti minimi brevis.

Roots C8-T1

Trunk Lower

Cord Medial

Nerve Ulnar

Open Chain Actions

SOLO ACTION
- Abduction of the metacarpophalangeal joint of digit 5

COMBINED ACTION
- Flexion of the metacarpophalangeal joint of digit 5
- Extension of interphalangeal joints via its insertion onto the dorsal expansion

Closed Chain Action N/A

Synergists

Muscle	Nerve	Root
• Interossei [47,48]	Ulnar	C8-T1
• Flexor digitorum profundus [37]	Anterior interosseus (median), ulnar	C7-T1
• Flexor digitorum superficialis [35]	Median	C7-T1
• Lumbricals, 4th [42]	Ulnar	C7-T1

Antagonists

Muscle	Nerve	Root
• Palmar intereossei [47]	Ulnar	C8-T1
• Extensor digitorum communis [26]	Posterior interosseus (radial)	C6-8
• Extensor digiti minimi	Posterior interosseus (radial)	C6-8

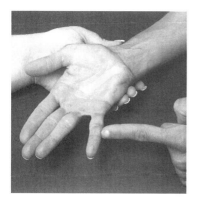

MUSCLE TESTING INSTRUCTIONS

Patient
Sitting or supine, the patient abducts the little finger.

Tester
The tester is in front of or to the side of the patient. With the hand stabilized, an adduction vector is generated against the ulnar aspect of the middle phalanx of the 5th digit.

Test
"Push your little finger out against me."

Pitfalls
N/A

CLINICAL PEARLS

N/A

45. FLEXOR DIGITI MINIMI

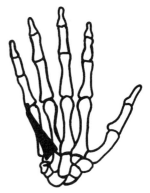

Origin
- Hamate bone
- Contiguous parts of the transverse carpal ligament

Insertion
- Ulnar side of the base of the proximal phalanx of the 5th digit

Roots C8-T1

Trunk Lower

Cord Medial

Nerve Ulnar

Open Chain Actions
SOLO ACTION
- Flexion of the metacarpophalangeal joint of digit 5

COMBINED ACTION
- Opposition of digit 5 to the thumb

Closed Chain Action N/A

Synergists

Muscle	Nerve	Root
• Opponens digiti minimi [43]	Ulnar	C8-T1
• Lumbricals 3 and 4 [42]	Ulnar	C7-T1
• Interossei [47, 48]	Ulnar	C8-T1
• Flexor digitorum profundus [37]	Ulnar	C7-T1
• Flexor digitorum superficialis 35]	Median	C7-T1

Antagonists

Muscle	Nerve	Root
• Extensor digitorum communis [26]	Posterior interosseus (radial)	C6-8
• Extensor digiti minimi	Posterior interosseus (radial)	C6-8

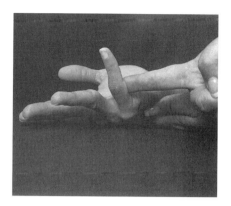

MUSCLE TESTING INSTRUCTIONS

Patient
Sitting or supine, the patient flexes the little finger.

Tester
The tester is in front of or to the side of the patient. An extension vector is generated against the flexed proximal phalanx of the 5th digit with the interphalangeal joints extended.

Test
"Push against my finger."

Pitfalls
N/A

CLINICAL PEARLS

N/A

46. ADDUCTOR POLLICIS

Origin
- Oblique head
  - Capitate bone
  - Bases of the 2d and 3d metacarpals
  - Intercarpal ligaments
- Transvere head
  - Proximal two-thirds of the palmar surface of the 3d metacarpal bone

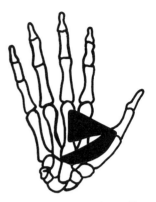

Insertion
- Oblique: Extensor expansion of the thumb
- Transverse: Medial surface of the base of the proximal phalanx of the thumb

Roots C8-T1

Trunk Lower

Cord Medial

Nerve Ulnar

Open Chain Actions
SOLO ACTION
- Adduction of the carpometacarpal joint of the thumb

COMBINED ACTION
- Adduction of the metacarpophalangeal joint of the thumb
- Flexion of the metacarpophalangeal joint of the thumb
- Assists in opposition of the thumb
- Extension of the interphalangeal joint of the thumb by way of its insertion into the extensor expansion

Closed Chain Action N/A

Synergists

Muscle	Nerve	Root
• Extensor pollicis longus [29]	Posterior interosseus (radial)	C6-8
• Flexor pollicis longus [36]	Anterior interosseus (median)	C7-T1
• Flexor pollicis brevis [41]	Median, ulnar	C7-T1
• Opponens pollicis [40]	Median	C7-T1
• 1st Palmar interosseus	Ulnar	C8-T1

Antagonists

Muscle	Nerve	Root
• Abductor pollicis brevis [39]	Median	C7-T1
• Abductor pollicis longus [30]	Posterior interosseus (radial)	C6-8
• Flexor pollicis longus [36]	Anterior interosseus (median)	C7-T1
• Extensor pollicis brevis [31]	Posterior interosseus (radial)	C6-8

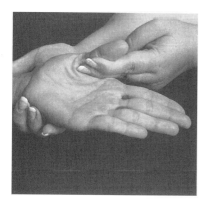

MUSCLE TESTING INSTRUCTIONS

Patient
Sitting or supine with the hand stabilized on the table by the tester, the patient approximates the thumb to the hand.

Tester
The tester is sitting or standing beside the patient and generates an abduction vector to the inner aspect of the thumb.

Test
"Push down against my fingers."

Pitfalls
N/A

CLINICAL PEARLS

1. The adductor pollicis [46] is the deepest of the thenar muscles.
2. With a strong adductor pollicis [46], the patient should be able to hold a piece of paper between the thumb and the index finger.
3. Contracture of this muscle leads to an adducton deformity of the thumb.
4. Some authors consider the first palmar interosseus [47] muscle to actually be a part of this muscle.

47. PALMAR INTEROSSEI

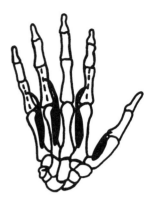

Origin

- 1st: Ulnar side of the base of the 1st metacarpal bone
- 2d: Ulnar side of the 2d metacarpal bone
- 3d: Radial side of the 4th metacarpal bone
- 4th: Radial side of the 5th metacarpal bone

Insertion

- Extensor expansion of the 2d, 4th, and 5th digits.
- Variable insertion into the proximal phalanx of the 2d digit (ulnar side), 4th digit (radial side), and 5th digit (radial side).
- First palmar interosseus blends with the adductor pollicis [46] to insert on the ulnar side of the proximal phalanx of the thumb (see Clinical Pearls).

Copyright © 1997, McGraw-Hill.

Roots C8-T1

Trunk Lower

Cord Medial

Nerve Ulnar

Open Chain Actions

Solo Action:
- Adduction of the 1st, 2d, 4th, and 5th digits toward the midline created by the 3d finger

Combined Action:
- Assists in flexion of the metacarpophalangeal joints
- Assists in extension of the interphalangeal joints

Closed Chain Action N/A

Synergists

Muscle	Nerve	Root
• Dorsal interossei [48]	Ulnar	C8-T1
• Lumbricals [42]	Median, ulnar	C7-T1
• Flexor digitorum profundus [37]	Anterior interosseus (median), ulnar	C7-T1
• Flexor digitorum superficialis [35]	Median	C7-T1
• Extensor indicis [28]	Posterior interosseus (radial)	C6-8
• Extensor digitorum communis [26]	Posterior interosseus (radial)	C6-8
• Extensor digiti minimi	Posterior interosseus (radial)	C6-8
• Abductor digiti minimi [44]	Ulnar	C8-T1
• Flexor digiti minimi [45]	Ulnar	C8-T1
• Opponens digiti minimi [43]	Ulnar	C8-T1
• Adductor pollicis [46]	Ulnar	C8-T1

Antagonists

Muscle	Nerve	Root
• Dorsal interossei [48]	Ulnar	C8-T1
• Extensor digitorum communis [26]	Posterior interosseus (radial)	C6-8
• Extensor indicis [28]	Posterior interosseus (radial)	C6-8
• Extensor digiti minimi	Posterior interosseus (radial)	C6-8
• Abductor digiti minimi [44]	Ulnar	C8-T1
• Flexor digitorum profundus [37]	Anterior interosseus (median), ulnar	C7-T1
• Flexor digitorum superficialis [35]	Median	C7-T1
• Lumbricals [42]	Median, ulnar	C7-T1

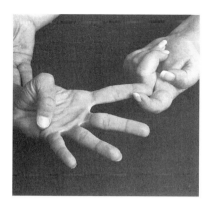

MUSCLE TESTING INSTRUCTIONS

Patient
Sitting or supine with the digits not being tested stabilized, the patient brings the finger toward the midline.

Tester
The tester is sitting or standing beside the patient, with the patient's hand in front of the tester. Pressure is generated in an abduction vector against the appropriate side of the distal phalanx of the thumb, index, ring, or little fingers.

Test
"Push your finger against mine."

Pitfalls
N/A

CLINICAL PEARLS

1. Some authors consider the first palmar interosseus [47] muscle to actually be a part of the adductor pollicis [46].
2. Contracture of the palmar interossei [47] results in the fingers held in an adducted position.
3. Weakness of the palmar interossei [47] may result in difficulty holding common objects such as a newspaper.
4. The student should remember the simple mnemonic: PAD = palmar interossei adduct.

48. DORSAL INTEROSSEI

Origin
- 1st lateral head: Ulnar side of the proximal portion of the 1st metacarpal bone.
  Medial head: Radial side of the 2d metacarpal bone
- 2d, 3d, and 4th: Interspace between the metacarpal bones.

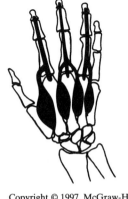

Insertion
- Base of the proximal phalanges of the radial side of the 2d
- Radial and ulnar sides of the 3d, and ulnar side of the 4th digits
- Expansion on the dorsum of the fingers

Roots C8-T1

Trunk Lower

Cord Medial

Nerve Ulnar

Open Chain Actions
SOLO ACTION
- Abduction of the 2d, 3d, and 5th fingers from the midline, which is through the 3d digit

COMBINED ACTION
- Assists in flexion of the metacarpophalangeal joints
- Assists in extension of the interphalangeal joints

Closed Chain Action N/A

Synergists

Muscle	Nerve	Root
• Lumbricals [42]	Median, ulnar	C7-T1
• Palmar interossei [47]	Ulnar	C8-T1
• Abductor digiti minimi [44]	Ulnar	C8-T1
• Flexor digiti minimi [45]	Ulnar	C8-T1
• Opponens digiti minimi [43]	Ulnar	C8-T1
• Flexor digitorum superficialis [35]	Median	C7-T1
• Flexor digitorum profundus [37]	Anterior interosseus (median), ulnar	C7-T1
• Extensor digitorum communis [26]	Posterior interosseus (radial)	C6-8
• Extensor indicis [28]	Posterior interosseus (radial)	C6-8
• Extensor digit minimi	Posterior interosseus (radial)	C6-8

Antagonists

Muscle	Nerve	Root
• Palmar interossei [47]	Ulnar	C8-T1
• Extensor digitorum communis [26]	Posterior interosseus (radial)	C6-8
• Extensor indicis [28]	Posterior interosseus (radial)	C6-8
• Extensor digit minimi	Posterior interosseus (radial)	C6-8
• Flexor digitorum superficialis [35]	Median	C7-T1
• Flexor digitorum profundus [37]	Anterior interosseus (median), ulnar	C7-T1

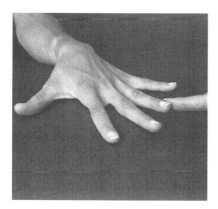

MUSCLE TESTING INSTRUCTIONS

Patient

Sitting or standing, with the digits not being tested stabilized, the patient moves the finger away from the midline.

Tester

The tester is sitting or standing beside the patient with the patient's hand in front of the tester. Pressure is generated against the distal phalanx of the appropriate digit in an adduction direction.

Test

"Push your finger against mine."

Pitfalls

N/A

CLINICAL PEARLS

1. The dorsal interossei [48] are four bipennate muscles lying between the five metacarpal bones at the back of the hand.
2. Marked contracture of the dorsal interossei [48] will result in abduction of digits 2 and 5.
3. Weakness of the dorsal interossei [48] may result in difficulty holding common objects such as a newspaper.
4. The student should remember the simple mnemonic: DAB = Dorsal interossei abduct.

49. PALMARIS BREVIS

Origin
- Palmar side of both the aponeurosis
- Flexor retinaculum along the ulnar border

Insertion
- Skin on palmar surface of the ulnar side of the hand

Roots C7-T1

Trunk Middle and lower

Cord Medial

Nerve Ulnar

Open Chain Actions
SOLO ACTION
- Wrinkles the skin on the ulnar aspect of the hand
COMBINED ACTION N/A

Closed Chain Action N/A

Synergists N/A

Antagonists N/A

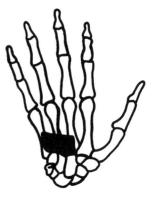

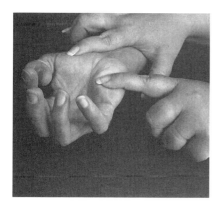

MUSCLE TESTING INSTRUCTIONS

Patient

Sitting or supine with the forearm resting on the table or bed in a supinated position, the patient cups or wrinkles the skin at the base of the hand.

Tester

The tester stands or sits in front of the patient, placing pressure against the thenar and hypothenar eminences in an attempt to flatten the palm of the hand. The skin on the ulnar side of the hand should be observed for wrinkling.

Test

"Try to cup your hand."

Pitfalls

N/A

CLINICAL PEARLS

1. This muscle is usually innervated by the superficial branch of the ulnar nerve.

50. FLEXOR CARPI ULNARIS

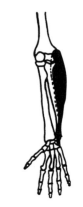

Origin
- Medial epicondyle of humerus (via common flexor tendon)
- Medial aspect of olecranon
- Proximal two-thirds of ulna
- Antebrachial fascia

Insertion:
- Hamate
- Fifth metacarpal
- Pisiform

Roots C8-T1

Trunk Lower

Cord Medial

Nerve Ulnar

Open Chain Actions
SOLO ACTION:
- Wrist flexion
- Wrist ulnar deviation

COMBINED ACTION:
- Elbow flexion

Closed Chain Action N/A

Synergists

Muscle	Nerve	Root
• Flexor carpi radialis [33]	Median	C6-8
• Palmaris longus [34]	Median	C7-T1
• Flexor digitorum profundus [37]	Anterior interosseus (median), ulnar	C7-T1
• Flexor digitorum superficialis [35]	Median	C7-T1
• Flexor pollicis longus [36]	Anterior interosseus (median)	C7-T1
• Extensor carpi ulnaris [27]	Radial	C6-8
• Biceps brachii [20]	Musculocutaneous	C5-6
• Brachialis [21]	Musculocutaneous, radial	C5-7
• Pronator teres [32]	Median	C6-7
• Brachioradialis [23]	Radial	C5-6
• Extensor carpi radialis longus and brevis [25]	Radial	C6-7

Antagonists

Muscle	Nerve	Root
• Triceps brachii and anconeus [22]	Radial	C6-8
• Extensor carpi radialis longus and brevis [25]	Radial	C6-7
• Extensor carpi ulnaris [27]	Radial	C6-8
• Extensor digitorum communis [26]	Radial	C6-8
• Extensor indicis [28]	Radial	C6-8
• Extensor digiti minimi	Radial	C6-8
• Extensor pollicis longus [29]	Radial	C6-8
• Flexor carpi radialis [33]	Median	C6-8
• Extensor pollicis brevis [31]	Radial	C6-8
• Abductor pollicis longus [30]	Radial	C6-8

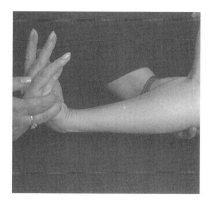

MUSCLE TESTING INSTRUCTIONS

Patient
Supine or sitting with the forearm supported, the wrist is flexed and fingers are relaxed. The patient flexes and ulnarly deviates the wrist.

Tester
The tester stabilizes the wrist and with the other hand generates a radial and extension vector.

Test
"Bring your wrist up and toward your body."

Pitfalls
N/A

CLINICAL PEARLS

1. This muscle is usually supplied by several twigs of the ulnar nerve, usually at or distal to the medial epicondyle of the elbow. This muscle is usually spared in cutibal tunnel syndrome.

QUESTIONS

1. Which muscles act to bring about interphalangeal joint flexion?
2. Which muscles of the forearm and hand have a dual innervation?
3. What are the different features in the muscle test of the pronator teres [32] and pronator quadratus [38]?
4. Name the muscles of the forearm and hand supplied by the posterior interosseus nerve.
5. Which muscles are involved in anterior interosseus syndrome?
6. What is the distal most muscle supplied by the radial nerve?
7. Name the boundaries of the "anatomic snuff box."
8. At the wrist, the median nerve usually lies between the tendons of which two muscles?
9. Describe the intrinsic "plus and minus" positions of the hand.
10. Holding a piece of paper between the thumb and index finger usually involves which muscles?

CHAPTER 5

HIP AND THIGH

Fae H. Garden and Carol Bodenheimer

Obturator externus
Quadratus femoris

MUSCLE FUNCTION AT SPECIFIC JOINTS

Hip flexion
Iliopsoas
Quadriceps (rectus femoris)
Pectineus
Tensor fascia lata
Gluteus minimus
Sartorius
Adductor longus
Adductor magnus (anterior part)
Adductor brevis
Gluteus medius

Hip extension
Gluteus maximus
Adductor magnus (posterior part)
Piriformis
Semimembranosus
Semitendinosus
Gluteus medius
Biceps femoris (long head)

Hip abduction
Gluteus medius
Gluteus minimus
Gluteus maximus (can assist in abduction when the hip is flexed)
Sartorius
Tensor fascia lata
Piriformis

Hip adduction
Adductor brevis
Pectineus
Adductor magnus
Gracilis
Gluteus maximus
Adductor longus
Iliopsoas

Hip internal rotation
Gluteus medius
Gluteus minimus
Tensor fascia lata
Semitendinosus
Semimembranosus

Hip external rotation
Gluteus maximus
Sartorius

Piriformis (as well as other small external rotator muscles of the hip, not mentioned in this book)

Gluteus medius

Iliopsoas

Biceps femoris (long head)

51. ILIOPSOAS

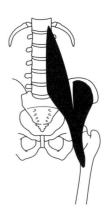

Origin
- Iliacus portion
  - Inner surface of the ilium
  - Internal lip of iliac crest
  - Iliolumbar ligaments
  - Ventral sacroiliac ligaments
  - Ala of sacrum
- Psoas portion
  - Anterolateral aspect of T12-L5 vertebral bodies
  - Transverse processes of T12-L5

Insertion
- Common insertion on and just distal to the lesser trochanter of the femur

Roots L2-L4

Trunk N/A

Cord N/A

Nerve
- Iliacus: femoral nerve
- Psoas: ventral rami of L2-4

Open Chain Actions
SOLO ACTION
- Hip flexion
- Hip external rotation
- Hip adduction

COMBINED ACTION N/A

Closed Chain Action Flexes the trunk toward the leg (e.g., in a supine-to-sit transfer)

Synergists

Muscle	Nerve	Root
• Sartorius [61]	Femoral	L2-4
• Pectineus [58]	Femoral	L2-4
• Tensor fascia lata [55]	Superior gluteal	L4-S1
• Adductor brevis and longus [56]	Obturator	L2-4
• Adductor magnus (anterior) [57]	Obturator	L2-4
• Gluteus minimus [54]	Superior gluteal	L4-S1
• Quadriceps (rectus femoris) [62]	Femoral	L2-4
• Adductor longus/brevis [56]	Obturator	L2-4
• Adductor magnus (anterior) [57]	Obturator	L2-4
• Gluteus medius [53]	Superior gluteal	L4-S1
• Gluteus maximus [52]	Inferior gluteal	L5-S2
• Piriformis [60]	Nerve to the piriformis	S1-2
• Biceps femoris (long head) [63]	Tibial division of sciatic	L5-S2
• Gracilis [59]	Obturator	L2-4

Antagonists

Muscle	Nerve	Root
• Erector spinae	Dorsal ram of spinal nerves	N/A
• Gluteus maximus [52]	Inferior gluteal	L5-S2
• Adductor magnus (posterior) [57]	Tibial division of sciatic	L4-S1
• Gluteus medius [53]	Superior gluteal	L4-S1
• Semimembranosus/semitendinosus [64]	Tibial division of sciatic	L5-S2
• Biceps femoris (long head) [63]	Tibial division of sciatic	L5-S2
• Piriformis [60]	Nerve to the piriformis	S1-2
• Gluteus minimus [54]	Superior gluteal	L4-S1
• Tensor fascia lata [55]	Superior gluteal	L4-S1
• Sartorius [61]	Femoral	L2-4

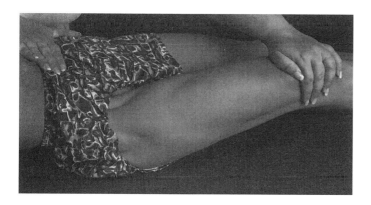

MUSCLE TESTING INSTRUCTIONS

Patient

Technique 1: Supine (on a firm surface) with the knee extended and the hip slightly abducted, the patient flexes the hip.

Technique 2: Sitting with knee flexed, the patient flexes the hip.

Tester

The tester applies pressure on the distal femur, in the vector of hip extension.

Test

"Lift your leg toward the ceiling" or "pick your leg up off the bed."

Pitfalls

Don't allow the patient to externally rotate the femur as this will cause the adductors to fire.

CLINICAL PEARLS

1. Lesions in the retroperitoneal space (e.g., hematoma, abscess) may contribute to clinical weakness in this muscle.
2. This muscle is the most powerful hip flexor.

52. GLUTEUS MAXIMUS

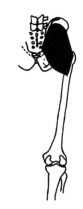

Origin
- Dorsal aspect of the sacrum
- Dorsal sacroiliac ligaments and sacrotuberous ligaments
- Lateral ilium near the posterior superior iliac spine

Insertion
- Upper fibers: lateral portion of the fascia lata (also called the iliotibial band)
- Lower fibers: gluteal tuberosity of the femur

Roots L5-S2

Trunk N/A

Cord N/A

Nerve Inferior gluteal

Open Chain Actions
SOLO ACTION
- Hip extension
- Hip external rotation
- Hip abduction (upper fibers)
- Hip adduction (lower fibers)

COMBINED ACTION N/A

Closed Chain Actions
- Extends the trunk away from the leg (in standing up from a bent position)
- Moves the femur from the flexed position to neutral (in sit to stand) or to the extended position (in stair climbing) (knee extension)

Synergists

Muscle	Nerve	Root
• Adductor magnus [57]	Obturator, tibial division of sciatic	L2-S1
• Gluteus medius [53]	Superior gluteal	L4-S1
• Semitendinosus/semimembranosus [64]	Tibial	L5-S2
• Biceps femoris (long head) [63]	Tibial division of sciatic	L5-S2
• Gluteus minimus [54]	Superior gluteal	L4-S1
• Tensor fascia lata [55]	Superior gluteal	L4-S1
• Piriformis [60]	Nerve to piriformis	S1-2
• Sartorius [61]	Femoral	L2-4
• Iliopsoas [51]	Femoral	L2-4
• Adductor brevis and longus [56]	Obturator	L2-4
• Pectineus [58]	Femoral	L2-4
• Gracilis [59]	Obturator	L2-4

Antagonists

Muscle	Nerve	Root
• Iliopsoas [51]	Femoral	L2-4
• Pectineus [58]	Femoral	L2-4
• Tensor fascia lata [55]	Superior gluteal	L4-S1
• Adductor brevis and longus [56]	Obturator	L2-4
• Adductor magnus [57]	Obturator, tibial division of obturator	L2-S1
• Gluteus minimus [54]	Superior gluteal	L4-S1
• Gluteus medius [53]	Superior gluteal	L4-S1
• Sartorius [61]	Femoral	L2-4
• Quadriceps (rectus femoris) [62]	Femoral	L2-4
• Semitendinosus/semimembranosus [64]	Tibial	L5-S2
• Gracilis [59]	Obturator	L2-4
• Piriformis [60]	Nerve to piriformis	S1-2

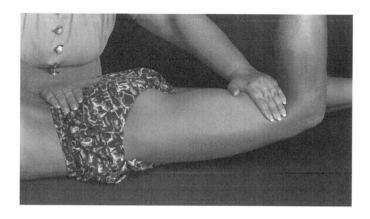

MUSCLE TESTING INSTRUCTIONS

Patient
Prone on a firm surface with the knee flexed to at least 90 degrees, the patient extends the hip.

Tester
The tester generates a flexion vector with downward pressure over the distal femur.

Test
"Pick your leg up."

Pitfalls
The knee must be flexed to at least 90 degrees so as to eliminate hamstring activation in hip extension.

CLINICAL PEARLS

1. This is the "power" extensor of the hip. It is activated, for example, during stair climbing or standing from a squatted or seated position, but not as much in normal gait.
2. If this muscle is severely weakened or absent, the characteristic lurching "gluteus maximus gait" may develop.

53. GLUTEUS MEDIUS

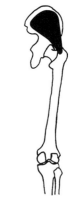

Origin
- Upper lateral surface of the wing of the ilium between the anterior and posterior lines

Insertion
- Greater trochanter of the femur

Roots L4-S1

Trunk N/A

Cord N/A

Nerve Superior gluteal

Open Chain Actions

SOLO ACTION:
- Hip abduction
- Hip flexion (anterior portion)
- Hip internal rotation (anterior portion)
- Hip extension (posterior portion)
- Hip external rotation (posterior portion)

COMBINED ACTION:
- Hip abduction
- Hip flexion (anterior portion)
- Hip internal rotation (anterior portion)
- Hip extension (posterior portion)
- Hip external rotation (posterior portion)

Closed Chain Actions:
- Lateral bending of the trunk
- Prevents the contralateral side of the pelvis from dropping during the stance phase of gait

Synergists

Muscle	Nerve	Root
• Gluteus minimus [54]	Superior gluteal	L4-S1
• Tensor fascia lata [55]	Superior gluteal	L4-S1
• Sartorius [61[	Femoral	L2-4
• Iliopsoas [51]	Femoral	L2-4
• Quadriceps (rectus femoris) [62]	Femoral	L2-4
• Pectineus [58]	Femoral	L2-4
• Adductor longus and brevis [56]	Obturator	L2-4
• Adductor magnus [57]	Obturator, tibial division of sciatic	L2-S1
• Gracilis [59]	Obturator	L2-4
• Semitendinosus/semimembranosus [64]	Tibial division of sciatic	L5-S2
• Gluteus maximus [52]	Inferior gluteal	L5-S2
• Piriformis [60]	Nerve to the piriformis	S1-2
• Biceps femoris (long head) [63]	Tibial of sciatic	L5-S2

Antagonists

Muscle	Nerve	Root
• Tensor fascia lata [55]	Superior gluteal	L4-S1
• Sartorius [61]	Femoral	L2-4
• Iliopsoas [51]	Femoral	L2-4
• Quadriceps (rectus femoris) [62]	Femoral	L2-4
• Pectineus [58]	Femoral	L2-4
• Adductor longus and brevis [56]	Obturator	L2-4
• Adductor magnus [57]	Obturator, tibial of sciatic	L2-S1
• Gracilis [59]	Obturator	L2-4
• Semitendinosus/semimembranosus [64]	Tibial	L5-S2
• Gluteus maximus [52]	Inferior gluteal	L5-S2
• Piriformis [60]	Nerve to the piriformis	S1-2
• Biceps femoris (long head) [63]	Tibial of sciatic	L5-S2
• Gluteus minimus [54]	Superior gluteal	L4-S1

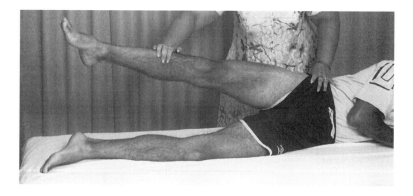

MUSCLE TESTING INSTRUCTIONS

Patient

Lying in the lateral position (contralateral side down) with the hip in slight extension and lateral rotation, the patient abducts the hip.

Tester

The tester generates a vector of adduction and minimal flexion of the hip to the distal femur.

Test

"Lift your leg up."

Pitfalls

If the hip is allowed to flex during this maneuver, hip flexors will also be tested. This is an inappropriate substitution.

CLINICAL PEARLS

1. This muscle is cut and reflected back in the posterolateral surgical approach for total hip arthroplasty.
2. Weakness in this muscle and the gluteus minimus [54] causes a Trendelenburg gait pattern.
3. Other muscles (sartorius [61], obturator internus, upper portion of gluteus maximus [52]) can abduct the femur in an open chain action, but only the gluteus medius [53] and minimus [54] can stabilize the pelvis in a closed chain action.
4. Electromyographic data have shown that this muscle is active in extension and external rotation but not in flexion and internal rotation, although it potentially has those actions.
5. The tester applying pressure in slight hip flexion helps differentiate this muscle from the gluteus minimus [54].

54. GLUTEUS MINIMUS

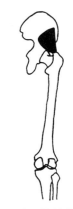

Origin
- Lateral surface of ilium between the anterior and posterior gluteal lines.

Insertion
- Greater trochanter of femur.

Roots L4-S1

Trunk N/A

Cord N/A

Nerve Superior gluteal

Open Chain Actions
SOLO ACTION
- Hip abduction
- Hip flexion
- Hip internal rotation

COMBINED ACTION
- Hip abduction
- Hip flexion
- Hip internal rotation

Closed Chain Actions
- Lateral bending of trunk
- Prevents the contralateral side of the pelvis from dropping in the stance phase of gait

Synergists

Muscle	Nerve	Root
• Gluteus medius [53]	Superior gluteal	L4-S1
• Tensor fascia lata [55]	Superior gluteal	L4-S1
• Sartorius [61]	Femoral	L2-4
• Iliopsoas [51]	Femoral	L2-4
• Quadriceps (rectus femoris) [62]	Femoral	L2-4
• Pectineus [58]	Femoral	L2-4
• Adductor longus and brevis [56]	Obturator	L2-4
• Adductor magnus (anterior) [57]	Obturator	L2-4
• Gracilis [59]	Obturator	L2-4
• Semitendinosus/semimembranosus [64]	Tibial	L5-S2
• Gluteus maximus [52]	Inferior gluteal	L5-S2
• Piriformis [60]	Nerve to the piriformis	S1-2

Antagonists

Muscle	Nerve	Root
• Adductor longus and brevis [56]	Obturator	L2-4
• Adductor magnus [57]	Obturator, tibial	L2-S1
• Gracilis [59]	Obturator	L2-4
• Sartorius [61]	Femoral	L2-4
• Iliopsoas [51]	Femoral	L2-4
• Semitendinosus/semimembranosus [64]	Tibial	L5-S2
• Gluteus maximus [52]	Inferior gluteal	L5-S2
• Piriformis [60]	Nerve to the piriformis	S1-2
• Biceps femoris (long head) [63]	Tibial of sciatic	L5-S2
• Pectineus [58]	Femoral	L2-4
• Gluteus medius [53]	Superior gluteal	L4-S1

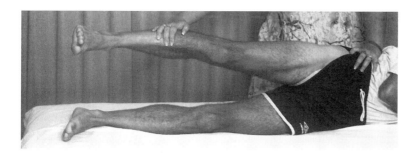

MUSCLE TESTING INSTRUCTIONS

Patient
Lying in the lateral position (contralateral side down), the patient abducts the hip avoiding any rotation, flexion or extension

Tester
Tester generates an adduction and minimal extension vector to the hip at the distal femur.

Test
"Lift your leg up."

Pitfalls
The hip joint should be in neutral antero-posterior position to test this muscle.

CLINICAL PEARLS

1. This muscle is cut and reflected back in the posterolateral surgical approach for total hip arthroplasty.
2. Weakness in the gluteus minimus [54] causes a Trendelenburg gait pattern.
3. Other muscles (sartorius [61], obturator internus, upper portion of gluteus maximus [52]) can abduct the femur in an open chain action but, only the gluteus medius [53] and minimus [54] can stabilize the pelvis in a closed chain action.
4. Electromyographic data show that this muscle is used in flexion and internal rotation but not in extension and external rotation, although it potentially has those actions.
5. The tester, applying pressure in slight extension, helps differentiate this muscle from the gluteus medius [53].

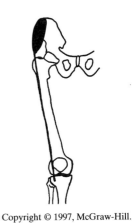

55. TENSOR FASCIA LATA

Origin
- Iliac crest just posterior to the anterior superior iliac spine

Insertion
- Iliotibial band at the junction of the proximal and middle thirds of the femur

Roots L4-S1

Trunk N/A

Cord N/A

Nerve Superior gluteal

Open Chain Actions
SOLO ACTION
- This muscle seldom acts alone. Please see its combined actions.

COMBINED ACTION
- Hip abduction in conjunction with the gluteus medius [53] and minimus [54]
- Hip flexion with the sartorius [61] and pectineus [58]
- Hip internal rotation especially with the anterior portion of the gluteus minimus [54]

Closed Chain Action Flexes the trunk toward the leg

Synergists

Muscle	Nerve	Root
• Iliopsoas [51]	Femoral	L2-4
• Sartorius [61]	Femoral	L2-4
• Pectineus [58]	Femoral	L2-4
• Gluteus medius [53]	Superior gluteal	L4-S1
• Gluteus minimus [54]	Superior gluteal	L4-S1
• Gracilis [59]	Obturator	L2-4
• Adductor brevis and longus [56]	Obturator	L2-4
• Adductor magnus (anterior) [57]	Obturator	L2-4
• Gluteus maximus [52]	Inferior gluteal	L5-S2
• Piriformis [60]	Nerve to the piriformis	S1-2
• Quadriceps (rectus femoris) [62]	Femoral	L2-4
• Semitendinosus/semimembranosus [64]	Tibial division of sciatic	L5-S2

Antagonists

Muscle	Nerve	Root
• Semitendinosus/semimembranosus [64]	Tibial	L5-S2
• Biceps femoris (long head) [63]	Tibial division of sciatic	L5-S2
• Gluteus medius [53]	Superior gluteal	L4-S1
• Adductor magnus [57]	Obturator, tibial division of sciatic	L2-S1
• Adductor brevis and longus [56]	Obturator	L2-4
• Pectineus [58]	Femoral	L2-4
• Gracilis [59]	Obturator	L2-4
• Gluteus maximus [52]	Inferior gluteal	L5-S2
• Piriformis [60]	Sciatic	S1-2
• Sartorius [61]	Femoral	L2-4
• Iliopsoas [51]	Femoral	L2-4
• Piriformis [60]	Nerve to the piriformis	S1-2

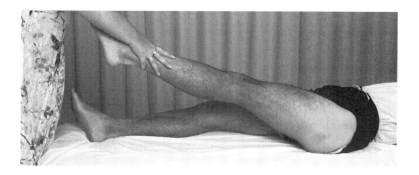

MUSCLE TESTING INSTRUCTIONS

Patient
Supine with the knee extended, the patient abducts, flexes, and internally rotates the hip.

Tester
The tester generates an extension vector on the distal femur.

Test
"Lift your leg up against my hand."

Pitfalls
N/A

CLINICAL PEARLS

1. Bilateral tightness of the tensor fascia lata [55] leads to an anterior pelvic tilt and perhaps bilateral genu valgus.
2. Unilateral tightness of the tensor fascia lata [55] may result in a lateral pelvic tilt and ipsilateral genu valgus. Bowlaged!
3. The tensor fascia lata [55] is functionally a "two-joint" muscle.

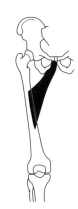

56. ADDUCTOR BREVIS AND LONGUS

Origin
- Adductor brevis: body and inferior ramus of pubic bone
- Adductor longus: pubic tubercle

Insertion
- Adductor brevis: pectineal line, proximal portion of linea aspera of the femur
- Adductor longus: medial edge of linea aspera of the femur

Roots L2-4

Trunk N/A

Cord N/A

Nerve Obturator

Open Chain Actions
SOLO ACTION
- Hip adduction

COMBINED ACTION
- Hip flexion

Closed Chain Action N/A

Synergists

Muscle	Nerve	Root
• Adductor magnus [57]	Obturator, tibial division of sciatic	L2-S1
• Gracilis [59]	Femoral	L2-4
• Iliopsoas [51]	Femoral	L2-4
• Quadriceps (rectus femoris) [62]	Femoral	L2-4
• Pectineus [58]	Femoral	L2-4
• Tensor fascia lata [55]	Superior gluteal	L4-S1
• Gluteus medius [53]	Superior gluteal	L4-S`
• Gluteus minimus [54]	Superior gluteal	L4-S1
• Sartorius [61]	Femoral	L2-4
• Gluteus maximus [52]	Inferior gluteal	L5-S2

Antagonists

Muscle	Nerve	Root
• Gluteus medius [53]	Superior gluteal	L4-S1
• Gluteus minimus [54]	Superior gluteal	L4-S1
• Tensor fascia lata [55]	Superior gluteal	L4-S1
• Gluteus maximus [52]	Inferior gluteal	L5-S2
• Semitendinosus/semimembranosus [64]	Tibial of sciatic	L5-S2
• Piriformis [60]	Nerve to the piriformis	S1-2
• Biceps femoris (long head) [63]	Tibial of sciatic	L5-S2
• Sartorius [61]	Femoral	L2-4
• Adductor magnus (posterior) [57]	Tibial division of sciatic	L4-S1

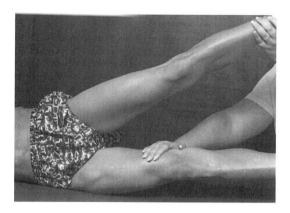

MUSCLE TESTING INSTRUCTIONS

Patient

Lying in the lateral position (ipsilateral side down), the patient adducts the ipsilateral hip so that the ipsilateral (bottom) limb lifts off the table.

Tester

The tester holds the contralateral (top) limb up and generates pressure to the ipsilateral distal femur in an abduction vector.

Test

"Raise your leg off the table."

Pitfalls

If the pelvis rotates forward during the test, the patient is using the gluteus maximus [52] for substitution. Flexion at the hip or anterior tilt of the pelvis allows for substitution by the hip flexors.

CLINICAL PEARLS

1. The hip adductors are tested as a group. Individual muscles cannot be isolated.
2. In testing the adductor group, when the muscle grade is 0 to 2, the patient should be supine and attempt to adduct the hip with no assistance or resistance by the examiner. Naturally, rotation must be avoided.

57. ADDUCTOR MAGNUS

Origin
- Inferior ramus of the pubic bone
- Ramus of the ischium
- Ischial tuberosity

Insertion
- Anterior fibers: linea aspera of the femur
- Posterior fibers: adductor tubercle of the femur

Roots
- Anterior portion: L2-4
- Posterior portion: L4-S1

Trunk N/A

Cord N/A

Nerve
- Anterior portion: obturator
- Posterior portion: tibial branch of the sciatic

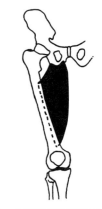

Open Chain Actions

SOLO ACTION
- Hip adduction
- Hip flexion (anterior fibers)
- Hip extension (posterior fibers)

COMBINED ACTION
- Anterior fibers flex the hip in combination with primary hip flexors
- Posterior fibers extend the hip in combination with primary hip extensors

Closed Chain Action N/A

Synergists

Muscle	Nerve	Root
• Adductor brevis and longus [56]	Obturator	L2-4
• Gracilis [59]	Obturator	L2-4
• Pectineus [58]	Femoral, obturator	L2-4
• Gluteus maximus [52]	Inferior gluteal	L5-S2
• Iliopsoas [51]	Femoral	L2-4
• Quadriceps (rectus femoris) [62]	Femoral	L2-4
• Tensor fascia lata [55]	Superior gluteal	L4-S1
• Gluteus medius [53]	Superior gluteal	L4-S1
• Gluteus minimus [54]	Superior gluteal	L4-S1
• Sartorius [61]	Femoral	L2-4
• Piriformis [60]	Nerve to the piriformis	S1-2
• Semitendinosus/semimembranosus [64]	Tibial of sciatic	L5-S2
• Biceps femoris (long head) [63]	Tibial divison of sciatic	L5-S2

Antagonists

Muscle	Nerve	Root
• Gluteus medius [53]	Superior gluteal	L4-S1
• Gluteus minimus [54]	Superior gluteal	L4-S1
• Tensor fascia lata [55]	Superior gluteal	L4-S1
• Sartorius [61]	Femoral	L2-4
• Gluteus maximus [52]	Inferior gluteal	L5-S2
• Iliopsoas [51]	Femoral	L2-4
• Quadriceps (rectus femoris) [62]	Femoral	L2-4
• Pectineus [58]	Femoral, obturator	L2-4
• Adductor brevis and longus [56]	Obturator	L2-4
• Piriformis [60]	Nerve to the piriformis	S1-2
• Semitendinosus/semimembranosus [64]	Tibial of sciatic	L5-S2
• Biceps femoris (long head) [63]	Tibial division of sciatic	L5-S2

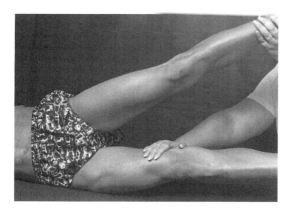

MUSCLE TESTING INSTRUCTIONS

Patient

Lying in the lateral position (ipsilateral side down), the patient adducts the ipsilateral hip so that the ipsilateral (bottom) limb lifts off the table.

Tester

The tester holds the contralateral (top) limb up and generates pressure to the ipsilateral distal femur in an abduction vector.

Test

"Raise your leg off the table."

Pitfalls

Do not allow the pelvis to roll forward, as the patient can substitute using the gluteus maximus [52]. Flexion at the hip or anterior tilt of the pelvis allows for substitution by the hip flexors.

CLINICAL PEARLS

1. The adductor magnus [57] has a dual nerve supply.
2. The hip adductors are tested as a group. Individual muscles cannot be isolated.
3. In testing the adductor group, when the muscle grade is 0 to 2, the patient should be supine and attempt to adduct the hip with no assistance or resistance by the examiner. Naturally, rotation must be avoided.

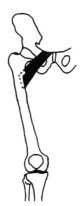

58. PECTINEUS

Origin
- Superior ramus of pubis (pectineal line)

Insertion
- Pectineal line on posterior surface of femur just distal to lesser trochanter

Roots L2-4

Trunk N/A

Cord N/A

Nerve
- Femoral nerve
- Accessory obturator if present or rarely the obturator nerve

Open Chain Actions
SOLO ACTION
- Hip flexion
- Hip adduction

COMBINED ACTION N/A

Closed Chain Action N/A

Synergists

Muscle	Nerve	Root
• Adductor longus and brevis [56]	Obturator	L2-4
• Adductor magnus [57]	Obturator, tibial division of sciatic	L2-S1
• Gracilis [59]	Obturator	L2-4
• Iliopsoas [51]	Femoral	L2-4
• Quadriceps (rectus femoris) [62]	Femoral	L2-4
• Tensor fascia lata [55]	Superior gluteal	L4-S1
• Gluteus minimus [54]	Superior gluteal	L4-S1
• Gluteus medius [53]	Superior gluteal	L4-S1
• Sartorius [61]	Femoral	L2-4
• Gluteus maximus [52]	Inferior gluteal	L5-S2

Antagonists

Muscle	Nerve	Root
• Gluteus medius [53]	Superior gluteal	L4-S1
• Gluteus minimus [54]	Superior gluteal	L4-S1
• Gluteus maximus [52]	Inferior gluteal	L5-S2
• Adductor magnus (posterior) [57]	Tibial division of sciatic	L5-S1
• Piriformis [60]	Nerve to the piriformis	S1-S2
• Semitendinosus/semimembranosus [64]	Tibial of sciatic	L5-S2
• Biceps femoris (long head) [63]	Tibial division of sciatic	L5-S2
• Tensor fascia lata [55]	Superior gluteal	L4-S1
• Sartorius [61]	Femoral	L2-4

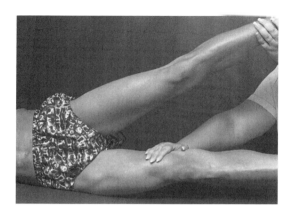

MUSCLE TESTING INSTRUCTIONS

Patient
Lying in the lateral position (ipsilateral side down), the patient adducts the ipsilateral hip so that the ipsilateral (bottom) limb lifts off the table.

Tester
The tester holds the contralateral (top) limb up and generates pressure to the ipsilateral distal femur in an abduction vector.

Test
"Raise your leg off the table."

Pitfalls
Do not allow the pelvis to roll forward, as the patient can substitute using the gluteus maximus [52]. Flexion at the hip or anterior tilt of the pelvis allows substitution by the hip flexors.

CLINICAL PEARLS

1. In testing the adductor group, when the muscle grade is 0 to 2, the patient should be supine and attempt to adduct the hip with no assistance or resistance by the examiner. Naturally, rotation must be avoided.
2. The pectineus [58] often has a dual nerve supply.
3. The hip adductors are tested as a group. Individual muscles cannot be isolated.

59. GRACILIS

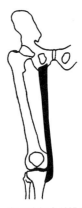

Origin
- Inferior pubic ramus

Insertion
- Proximal end of tibia, just distal to the medial epicondyle and proximal to the insertion of the semitendinosus [64] and lateral to the insertion of the sartorius [61] (pes anserine)

Roots L2-4

Trunk N/A

Cord N/A

Nerve Obturator

Open Chain Actions
SOLO ACTION
- Hip adduction
- Knee flexion
- Knee internal rotation

COMBINED ACTION
- When the knee is extended, it is technically possible for the gracilis [59] to flex the hip in combination with the hip flexors. However, this function is so weak that the gracilis [59] is not listed as a hip flexor in this chapter and is thus not included in the Synergists/Antagonists lists for this function.
- When the knee is flexed, it is technically possible for the gracilis [59] to internally rotate the hip in combination with the hip internal rotators. However, this function is so weak that the gracilis [59] is not listed as an internal rotator in this chapter and is thus not included in the Synergists/Antagonists lists for this function.

Closed Chain Action Flexes the trunk toward the femur

Synergists

Muscle	Nerve	Root
Adductor magnus [57]	Obturator, tibial division of sciatic	L2-S1
Adductor longus and brevis [56]	Obturator	L2-4
Pectineus [58]	Femoral	L2-4
Gluteus maximus [52]	Inferior gluteal	L5-S2
Iliopsoas [51]	Femoral	L2-4
Semitendinosus/semimembranosus [64]	Tibial division of sciatic	L5-S2
Biceps femoris [63]	Tibial and peroneal divisions of sciatic	L5-S2
Sartorius [61]	Femoral	L2-4
Gastrocnemius [72]	Tibial	L5-S2
Popliteus [65]	Tibial	L4-S1
Tensor fascia lata [55]	Superior gluteal	L4-S1

Antagonists

Muscle	Nerve	Root
Gluteus medius [53]	Superior gluteal	L4-S1
Gluteus minimus [54]	Superior gluteal	L4-S1
Tensor fascia lata [55]	Superior gluteal	L4-S1
Gluteus maximus [52]	Inferior gluteal	L5-S2
Sartorius [61]	Femoral	L2-4
Piriformis [60]	Nerve to the piriformis	S1-2
Quadriceps [62]	Femoral	L2-4
Biceps femoris [63]	Tibial and peroneal divisions of sciatic	L5-S2

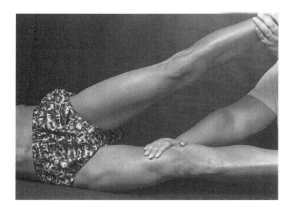

MUSCLE TESTING INSTRUCTIONS

Patient

Lying in the lateral position (ipsilateral side down), the patient adducts the ipsilateral hip so that the ipsilateral (bottom) limb lifts off the table.

Tester

The tester holds the contralateral (top) limb up and generates pressure to the ipsilateral distal femur in an abduction vector.

Test

"Raise your leg off the table."

Pitfalls

Do not allow the pelvis to roll forward as the patient can substitute using the gluteus maximus [52]. Flexion at the hip or anterior tilt of the pelvis allows substitution by the hip flexors.

CLINICAL PEARLS

1. In testing the adductor group, when the muscle grade is 0 to 2, the patient should be supine and attempt to adduct the hip with no assistance or resistance by the examiner. Naturally, rotation must be avoided.
2. The hip adductors are tested as a group. Individual muscles cannot be isolated.

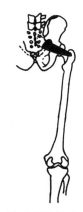

60. HIP ROTATORS (PIRIFORMIS)

Origin
- Pelvic surface of sacrum

Insertion
- Superior border of the greater trochanter of the femur

Roots S1-2

Trunk N/A

Cord N/A

Nerve Sacral plexus (nerve to the piriformis)

Open Chain Actions
SOLO ACTION
- Hip external rotation

COMBINED ACTION
- Hip extension
- Hip abduction

Closed Chain Action N/A

Synergists

Muscle	Nerve	Root
• Quadratus femoris	Nerve to the quadratus femoris	L4-S2
• Obturator internus	Nerve to the obturator internus	L5-S1
• Obturator externus	Obturator	L2-4
• Gemellus superior	Sacral plexus	L5-S2
• Gemellus inferior	Sacral plexus	L4-S1
• Gluteus maximus [52]	Inferior gluteal	L5-S2
• Iliopsoas [51]	Femoral	L2-4
• Biceps femoris (long head) [63]	Tibial division of sciatic	L5-S2
• Gluteus medius [53]	Superior gluteal	L4-S1
• Sartorius [61]	Femoral	L2-4
• Gluteus minimus [54]	Superior gluteal	L4-S1
• Tensor fascia lata [55]	Superior gluteal	L4-S1
• Adductor magnus (posterior) [57]	Tibial division of sciatic	L5-S1
• Semitendinosus/semimembranosus [64]	Tibial division of sciatic	L5-S2

Antagonists

Muscle	Nerve	Root
• Gluteus minimus [54]	Superior gluteal	L4-S1
• Tensor fasciae latae [55]	Superior gluteal	L4-S1
• Gracilis [59]	Obturator	L2-4
• Adductor brevis and longus [56]	Obturator	L2-4
• Adductor magnus [57]	Obturator, tibial of sciatic	L2-S1
• Pectineus [58]	Femoral, obturator	L2-4
• Semitendinosus/semimembranosus [64]	Tibial	L5-S2
• Gluteus medius [53]	Superior gluteal	L4-S1
• Gluteus maximus [52]	Inferior gluteal	L5-S2
• Iliopsoas [51]	Nerve to iliopsoas	L2-4
• Quadriceps (rectus femoris) [62]	Femoral	L2-4
• Sartorius [61]	Femoral	L2-4

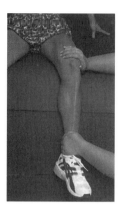

MUSCLE TESTING INSTRUCTIONS

Patient

Short sitting with the knees flexed, the patient rotates the hip laterally such that the foot moves toward the contralateral side.

Tester

The tester stabilizes the thigh by applying pressure distally and laterally in order to prevent abduction. With the other hand, the tester generates an internal rotation vector of the hip by applying pressure to the inner aspect of the leg.

Test

"Rotate your thigh outward against my hand."

Pitfalls

Suboptimal strength testing may result from buttock pain secondary to the "piriformis syndrome" or other similar maladies.

CLINICAL PEARLS

1. In a small percentage of cases, the sciatic nerve passes between the heads of the piriformis [60] muscle.

61. SARTORIUS

Origin
- Anterior superior iliac spine

Insertion
- Proximal part of the medial surface of the tibia just distal to the tibial condyle (pes anserine)

Roots L2-4

Trunk N/A

Cord N/A

Nerve Femoral

Open Chain Actions

SOLO ACTION
- Hip flexion
- Knee flexion
- Hip abduction
- Hip external rotation

COMBINED ACTION
- Assists in internal rotation of the knee along with the semimembranosus [64], semitendinosus [64], gracilis [59], and popliteus [65]

Closed Chain Action N/A

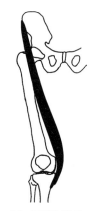

Synergists

Muscle	Nerve	Root
• Iliopsoas [51]	Femoral	L2-4
• Pectineus [58]	Femoral, obturator	L2-4
• Tensor fascia lata [55]	Superior gluteal	L4-S1
• Adductor brevis and longus [56]	Obturator	L2-4
• Semitendinosus/semimembranosus [64]	Tibial	L5-S2
• Biceps femoris [63]	Tibial, peroneal	L5-S2
• Gracilis [59]	Obturator	L2-4
• Quadriceps (rectus femoris) [62]	Femoral	L2-4
• Gluteus minimus [54]	Superior gluteal	L4-S1
• Adductor magnus [57]	Obturator, tibial division of sciatic	L2-S1
• Gluteus medius [53]	Superior gluteal	L4-S1
• Popliteus [65]	Tibial	L4-S1
• Gastrocnemius [72]	Tibial	L5-S2
• Gluteus maximus [52]	Inferior gluteal	L5-S2
• Piriformis [60]	Nerve to the piriformis	S1-2

Antagonists

Muscle	Nerve	Root
• Gluteus maximus [52]	Inferior gluteal	L5-S2
• Adductor magnus [57]	Obturator, tibial divison of sciatic	L2-S1
• Quadriceps [62]	Femoral	L2-4
• Piriformis [60]	Nerve to the piriformis	S1-2
• Semitendinosus/semimembranosus [64]	Tibial	L5-S2
• Gluteus medius [53]	Superior gluteal	L4-S1
• Biceps femoris [63]	Peroneal, tibial divisions of sciatic	L5-S2
• Adductor brevis and longus [56]	Obturator	L2-4
• Pectineus [58]	Femoral, obturator	L2-4
• Gracilis [59]	Obturator	L2-4
• Iliopsoas [51]	Femoral	L2-4
• Tensor fascia lata [55]	Superior gluteal	L4-S1

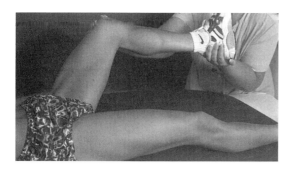

MUSCLE TESTING INSTRUCTIONS

Patient
Supine, the patient externally rotates, abducts, and flexes the hip while flexing the knee.

Tester
The tester creates an extension, internal rotation and adduction vector to the hip by generating pressure against the outer aspect of the distal thigh. Simultaneously, the other hand provides an extension vector to the knee.

Test
"Turn your thigh outward and bend your hip and knee."

Pitfalls
The sartorius [61] is a weak muscle with a large range of actions that can be duplicated by other lower limb muscles. The examiner must provide a combined resistance movement to test the multiple actions of the sartorius [61]. Isolated sartorius [61] testing can be technically difficult.

CLINICAL PEARLS

1. The sartorius [61] received its name, "the tailor muscle," because it helps initiate the action of crossing the legs.
2. The sartorius [61] is a two-joint muscle.

62. QUADRICEPS (RECTUS FEMORIS, VASTUS LATERALIS, MEDIALIS, INTERMEDIUS)

Origin
- Vastus lateralis
  - Linea aspera of femur
  - Greater trochanter of femur
  - Intertrochanteric line of femur
- Vastus medialis
  - Linea aspera of femur
  - Intertrochanteric line of femur
  - Tendons of adductor magnus and longus
- Vastus intermedius
  - Femur (upper two-thirds of the shaft)
- Rectus femoris: the two heads (tendons) conjoin to form an aponeurosis from which the muscle fibers arise
  - Straight head: anterior inferior iliac spine
  - Reflected head: groove above rim of acetabulum

Insertion:
- Proximal border of patella
- Tibial tuberosity through the patellar ligament

Roots L2-4

Trunk N/A

Cord N/A

Nerve Femoral

Open Chain Actions
SOLO ACTION:
- Extension of the knee joint
- Hip flexion (rectus femoris)

COMBINED ACTION:
- Assists in flexion of the hip

Closed Chain Action Responsible for controlling lowering of the body during a deep knee bend (eccentric knee flexion)

Synergists

Muscle	Nerve	Root
• Gluteus maximus [52]	Inferior gluteal	L5-S2
• Tensor fascia lata [55]	Superior gluteal	L4-S1
• Iliopsoas [51]	Femoral	L2-4
• Pectineus [58]	Femoral, obturator	L2-4
• Gluteus minimus [54]	Superior gluteal	L4-S1
• Gluteus medius [53]	Superior gluteal	L4-S1
• Sartorius [61]	Femoral	L2-4
• Adductor brevis and longus [56]	Obturator	L2-4
• Adductor magnus (anterior) [57]	Obturator	L2-4

Antagonists

Muscle	Nerve	Root
• Semitendinosus/semimembranosus [64]	Tibial	L5-S2
• Biceps femoris [63]	Tibial, peroneal divisions of sciatic	L5-S2
• Gracilis [59]	Obturator	L2-L4
• Sartorius [61]	Femoral	L2-L4
• Popliteus [65]	Tibial	L4-S1
• Gastrocnemius [72]	Tibial	L5-S2
• Tensor fascia lata [55]	Superior gluteal	L4-S1
• Gluteus maximus [52]	Inferior gluteal	L5-S2
• Adductor magnus (posterior) [57]	Tibial division of sciatic	L5-S1
• Piriformis [60]	Nerve to the piriformis	S1-2
• Gluteus medius [53]	Superior gluteal	L4-S1

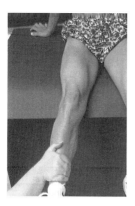

MUSCLE TESTING INSTRUCTIONS

Patient

Sitting at the edge of the table with the knees flexed, the patient leans backward to relax the hamstrings. The patient then straightens the knee.

Tester

The tester stands beside the patient and places one hand under the patient's thigh and the other over the anterior surface of the distal leg just proximal to the ankle. Resistance is applied in a flexion vector.

Test

"Straighten your leg."

Pitfalls

Hyperextension of the knee by the patient will "lock" the joint into position, giving an untrue strength test. Therefore in muscle testing, resistance should only be generated with the knee "unlocked."

CLINICAL PEARLS

1. Weakness of this muscle group will impair the ability to climb stairs, walk up an incline or stand from a seated position.
2. Prolonged weakness of the quadriceps [62] may result in knee hyperextension (genu recurvatum) during stance.
3. The superficial fibers of this muscle are bipennate but the deep fibers are parallel.
4. If the rectus femoris [62] is short, there can be restriction of knee flexion when the hip is extended or restriction of hip extension when the knee is flexed.
5. The genu articularis, a small muscle lying deep to the quadriceps, pulls the articular capsule proximally. This muscle cannot be clinically isolated.
6. The rectus femoris [62] is a "two-joint muscle."

63. BICEPS FEMORIS (SHORT AND LONG HEADS)

Origin
- Long head:
  - Inferior and medial aspects of the ischial tuberosity
  - Distal part of the sacrotuberous ligament
- Short head:
  - Linea aspera of the femur
  - Proximal part of the lateral supracondylar line
  - Lateral intermuscular septum

Insertion
- Lateral aspect of the fibular head
- Lateral condyle of the tibia
- Fascia on the lateral side of the leg
- Aponeurosis covering the muscle

Roots L5-S2

Trunk N/A

Cord N/A

Nerve: • Long head: sciatic (tibial division)   • Short head: sciatic (peroneal division)

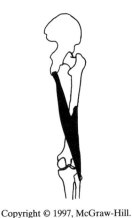

Open Chain Actions
SOLO ACTION:
- Long head:
  - Hip extension
  - Knee flexion
- Short head:
  - Knee flexion

COMBINED ACTION
- The long and short heads participate in external rotation of the knee
- The long head contributes to external rotation of the hip

Closed Chain Action During the gait cycle at heel strike, the hamstrings (biceps femoris [63], semitendinosus [64], and semimembranosus [64]) contract to assist in propelling the body forward.

Synergists

Muscle	Nerve	Root
• Gluteus maximus [52]	Inferior gluteal	L5-S2
• Gastrocnemius [72]	Tibial	L5-S2
• Tensor fascia lata [55]	Superior gluteal	L4-S1
• Semitendinosus/semimembranosus [64]	Tibial division of sciatic	L5-S2
• Adductor magnus (posterior) [57]	Tibial division of sciatic	L5-S1
• Piriformis [60]	Nerve to the piriformis	S1-2
• Gluteus medius [53]	Superior gluteal	L4-S1
• Gastrocnemius [72]	Tibial	L5-S2
• Gracilis [59]	Obturator	L2-4
• Sartorius [61]	Femoral	L2-4
• Popliteus [65]	Tibial	L4-S1
• Iliopsoas [51]	Femoral	L2-4

Antagonists

Muscle	Nerve	Root
• Quadriceps [62]	Femoral	L2-4
• Iliopsoas [51]	Femoral	L2-4
• Pectineus [58]	Femoral, obturator	L2-4
• Tensor fascia lata [55]	Superior gluteal	L4-S1
• Gluteus minimus [54]	Superior gluteal	L4-S1
• Gluteus medius [53]	Superior gluteal	L4-S1
• Sartorius [61]	Femoral	L2-4
• Adductor brevis and longus [56]	Obturator	L2-4
• Adductor magnus (anterior) [57]	Obturator	L2-4
• Semitendinosus/semimembranosus [64]	Sciatic (tibial)	L5-S2
• Gracilis [59]	Obturator	L2-4
• Popliteus [65]	Tibial	L4-S1

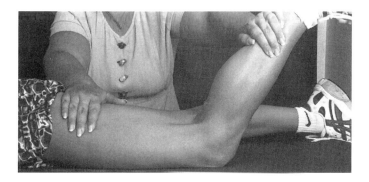

MUSCLE TESTING INSTRUCTIONS

Patient
Prone, the patient bends the knee.

Tester
After the patient has demonstrated full active range of motion, the tester holds the hip in a position of slight external rotation. The knee should also be slightly externally rotated on the thigh, i.e., toes point out. The knee should be in 30 to 45 degrees flexion in order to facilitate an accurate test. The examiner places pressure against the leg proximal to the ankle in order to resist knee flexion.

Test
"Pull your leg up."

Pitfalls
Testing this muscle in full flexion may be very uncomfortable for the patient.

CLINICAL PEARLS

1. The short head is sometimes absent
2. If the ipsilateral hip flexes when the knee has completed flexion, the tester should suspect a tight rectus femoris [62] muscle.
3. There are numerous muscles that can substitute for the hamstrings, e.g., the hip flexors, gracilis [59], sartorius [61], and gastrocnemius [72].
4. The short head of the biceps femoris [63] should always be tested electrodiagnostically when suspecting a peroneal neuropathy at the fibular head.
5. The biceps femoris [63] is a dually innervated muscle.

64. SEMITENDINOSUS AND SEMIMEMBRANOSUS

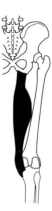

Origin
- Semitendinosus: ischial tuberosity (common tendon with long head of biceps femoris [63])
- Semimembranosus: ischial tuberosity (proximal and lateral to semitendinosus [64] and biceps femoris [63])

Insertion
- Semitendinosus
  - Proximal, medial aspect of the tibial shaft
  - Deep fascia of leg
- Semimembranosus
  - Posteromedial aspect of the medial condyle of the tibia

Roots L5-S2
Trunk N/A
Cord N/A
Nerve Sciatic (tibial division)
Open Chain Actions
SOLO ACTION
- Knee flexion
- Hip extension

COMBINED ACTION
- Assists in internal rotation of the hip joint
- Assists in internal rotation of the knee joint

Closed Chain Action
During the gait cycle at heel strike, the hamstrings (biceps femoris [63], semitendinosus [64], and semimembranosus [64]) contract to assist in propelling the body forward.

Synergists

Muscle	Nerve	Root
• Gluteus maximus [52]	Inferior gluteal	L5-S2
• Gastrocnemius [72]	Tibial	L5-S2
• Tensor fascia lata [55]	Superior gluteal	L4-S1
• Biceps femoris [63]	Tibial and peroneal divisions of sciatic	L5-S2
• Gracilis [59]	Obturator	L2-4
• Sartorius [61]	Femoral	L2-4
• Popliteus [65]	Tibial	L4-S1
• Adductor magnus (posterior) [57]	Tibial division of sciatic	L5-S1
• Piriformis [60]	Nerve to the piriformis	S1-2
• Gluteus medius [53]	Superior gluteal	L4-S1
• Gluteus minimus [54]	Superior gluteal	L4-S1

Antagonists

Muscle	Nerve	Root
• Quadriceps [62]	Femoral	L2-4
• Iliopsoas [51]	Femoral	L2-4
• Pectineus [58]	Femoral, obturator	L2-4
• Tensor fascia lata [55]	Superior gluteal	L4-S1
• Gluteus medius [53]	Superior gluteal	L4-S1
• Gluteus minimus [54]	Superior gluteal	L4-S1
• Sartorius [61]	Femoral	L2-4
• Adductor brevis and longus [56]	Obturator	L2-4
• Adductor magnus (anterior) [57]	Obturator	L2-4
• Gluteus maximus [52]	Inferior gluteal	L5-S2
• Piriformis [60]	Nerve to the piriformis	S1-2
• Biceps femoris [63]	Tibial and peroneal divisions of sciatic	L5-S2

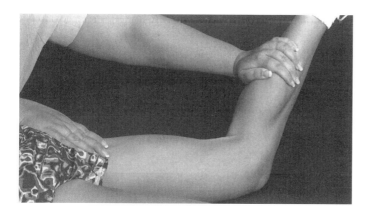

MUSCLE TESTING INSTRUCTIONS

Patient

Prone, the patient bends the knee.

Tester

After the patient has demonstrated full active range of motion, the tester holds the hip in a position of slight internal rotation. The knee should also be internally rotated, i.e., toes point in. The knee should be in 30 to 45 degrees flexion in order to facilitate a true test. The examiner places pressure against the leg proximal to the ankle in order to resist knee flexion.

Test

"Pull your leg up."

Pitfalls

Testing this muscle in full flexion may be uncomfortable for the patient.

CLINICAL PEARLS

1. The semitendinosus [64] and semimembranosus [64] are "two-joint muscles."
2. If the ipsilateral hip flexes when the knee has completed flexion, the tester should suspect a tight rectus femoris [62] muscle.

65. POPLITEUS

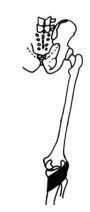

Origin
- Lateral condyle of the femur
- Lateral meniscus of knee
- From the arcuate ligament
- Part of the capsule of the knee joint

Insertion
- Posterior surface of proximal one-third of the tibia

Roots L4-S1

Trunk N/A

Cord N/A

Nerve Tibial

Open Chain Actions
SOLO ACTION
- Medial rotation of the tibia on the femur

COMBINED ACTION
- Knee flexion

Closed Chain Actions
- External rotation of the femur upon the tibia (distal fixation)
- Flexion of the knee

Synergists

Muscle	Nerve	Root
• Semimembranosus/semitendinosus [64]	Tibial	L5-S2
• Gracilis [59]	Obturator	L2-4
• Sartorius [61]	Femoral	L2-4
• Biceps femoris [63]	Tibial, peroneal division of sciatic	L5-S2
• Gastrocnemius [72]	Tibial	L5-S2
• Tensor fascia lata [55]	Superior gluteal	L4-S1

Antagonists

Muscle	Nerve	Root
• Biceps femoris [63]	Tibial, peroneal divisions of sciatic	L5-S2
• Quadriceps [62]	Femoral	L2-4

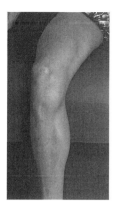 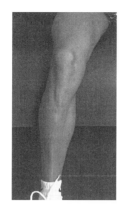

MUSCLE TESTING INSTRUCTIONS

Patient
Sitting with knee flexed at 90 degrees, the patient rotates the tibia medially

Tester
The popliteus [65] is tested to determine if the muscle is active and not to determine strength grade. Resistance is not generated by the tester (this is a "hands-off" test).

Test
"Keeping your thigh straight, try to turn your lower leg inward."

Pitfalls
N/A

CLINICAL PEARLS

1. In the gait cycle, this muscle is important in "unlocking the knee" in order to transition from stance to swing phase.

QUESTIONS

1. During what common activity is the gluteus maximus [52] active?
2. What substitution patterns does one need to avoid during testing of the adductor group?
3. What two nerves innervate the adductor magnus [57]?
4. What muscle insertions contribute to the pes anserine (and are involved in anserine bursitis)?
5. How is a patient positioned to test the tensor fascia lata [55]?
6. What is the primary (solo) action of the piriformis [60] muscle?
7. Name two joints that are simultaneously flexed by the sartorius muscle [61].
8. Which muscle combines with the quadriceps [62] group to assist with knee extension?
9. The long head of the biceps femoris [62] is innervated by which branch of the sciatic nerve?
10. Which muscles act to provide medial rotation of the tibia on the femur?

CHAPTER 6

LEG AND FOOT

Cliff A. Gronseth

MUSCLE FUNCTION AT SPECIFIC JOINTS

Knee flexion
Semitendinosus
Semimembranosus
Biceps femoris
Gracilis
Sartorius
Gastrocnemius
Popliteus
Tensor fascia lata

Knee extension
Quadriceps femoris
Gluteus maximus (via iliotibial band)

Knee internal rotation
Semitendinosus
Semimembranosus
Popliteus
Gracilis
Sartorius

Knee external rotation
Biceps femoris

Ankle dorsiflexion
Tibialis anterior
Peroneus tertius
Extensor hallucis longus
Extensor digitorum longus

Ankle plantarflexion
Gastrocnemius
Soleus
Flexor digitorum longus
Flexor hallucis longus
Tibialis posterior
Peroneus longus and brevis

Inversion
Tibialis anterior
Tibialis posterior
Flexor digitorum longus
Flexor hallucis longus
Extensor hallucis longus
Gastrocnemius (via the Achilles tendon)
Soleus (via the Achilles tendon)

Eversion
Peroneus longus and brevis
Peroneus tertius
Extensor digitorum longus

Toe flexion

      Flexor digitorum longus

      Lumbricales

      Dorsal interossei

      Plantar interossei

Toe extension

      Extensor digitorum longus

      Extensor digitorum brevis

Great toe flexion

      Flexor hallucis longus

      Abductor hallucis

Great toe extension

      Extensor hallucis longus

      Extension digitorum brevis

66. TIBIALIS ANTERIOR

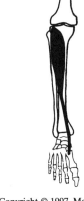

Origin
- Lateral condyle of the tibia
- Proximal one-half of the lateral surface of the tibia
- Interosseus membrane
- Deep fascia
- Lateral intermuscular septum

Insertion
- Medial and plantar surface of the medial cuneiform
- Base of the first metatarsal

Roots L4-S1

Nerve Deep peroneal

Open Chain Actions
Solo Action
- Ankle dorsiflexion
- Foot inversion

Combined Action
- Ankle dorsiflexion at midline with peroneii so as to balance

Closed Chain Action Tilts the leg forward when the foot is fixed and flexes the knee

Synergists

Muscle	Nerve	Root
• Extensor digitorum longus [67]	Deep peroneal	L4-S1
• Extensor hallucis longus [68]	Deep peroneal	L4-S1
• Peroneus tertius [69]	Deep peroneal	L4-S1
• Tibialis posterior [76]	Tibial	L5-S1
• Flexor digitorum longus [74]	Tibial	L5-S1
• Flexor hallucis longus [75]	Tibial	L5-S2
• Gastrocnemius [72]	Tibial	L5-S2
• Soleus [73]	Tibial	L5-S2

Antagonists

Muscle	Nerve	Root
• Tibialis posterior [76]	Tibial	L5-S1
• Peroneus longus and brevis [71]	Superficial peroneal	L4-S1
• Gastrocnemius [72]	Tibial	L5-S2
• Soleus [73]	Tibial	L5-S2
• Flexor digitorum longus [74]	Tibial	L5-S1
• Flexor hallucis longus [75]	Tibial	L5-S2
• Peroneus tertius [69]	Deep peroneal	L4-S1
• Extensor digitorum longus [67]	Deep peroneal	L4-S1

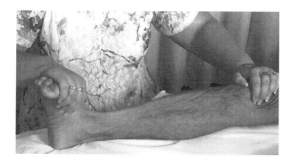

MUSCLE TESTING INSTRUCTIONS

Patient
The patient dorsiflexes and inverts the foot, without great toe extension.

Tester
The tester generates pressure on the medial and dorsal foot in an inferior/lateral direction. The other hand is placed on the lateral ankle/distal leg to counteract the ankle torque.

Test
"Push your foot against my hand by pointing your foot toward your nose."

Pitfalls
Counterforce must be generated on the lateral distal leg to stabilize the limb. Note that the extensor hallucis longus [68] can dorsiflex the ankle; therefore, when testing the tibialis anterior [66], the great toe should be pointed down.

CLINICAL PEARLS

1. A quick assessment of "functional strength" is to have the patient walk on the outside edge of the feet or on the heels. Look for symmetry of foot inversion.
2. The tibialis anterior [66] is the first large tendon palpated anterior to the medial malleolus.

67. EXTENSOR DIGITORUM LONGUS

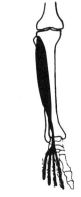

Origin

- Lateral condyle of the tibia
- Proximal three-quarters of the anterior surface of the body of the fibula
- Proximal part of the interosseus membrane
- Adjacent intermuscular septa
- Deep fascia

Insertion

- Extensor expansions into the middle and distal phalanges of the lateral four toes

Roots L4-S1

Nerve Deep peroneal

Open Chain Actions

SOLO ACTION

- Extension of the metatarsophalangeal joint of the lateral four toes
- Extension of the distal interphalangeal and proximal interphalangeal joints of the lateral four toes

COMBINED ACTION

- Ankle dorsiflexion
- Foot eversion

Closed Chain Action Tilts the leg forward when the foot is fixed and flexes the knee

Synergists

Muscle	*Nerve*	*Root*
• Extensor digitorum brevis [70]	Deep peroneal	L5-S1
• Extensor hallucis longus [68]	Deep peroneal	L4-S1
• Tibialis anterior [66]	Deep peroneal	L4-S1
• Peroneus tertius [69]	Deep peroneal	L4-S1
• Peroneus longus and brevis [71]	Superficial peroneal	L4-S1

Antagonists

Muscle	*Nerve*	*Root*
• Flexor digitorum longus [74]	Tibial	L5-S1
• Lumbricales [78]	Medial and lateral plantar (tibial)	L5-S2
• Plantar interossei [79]	Lateral plantar (tibial)	S1-2
• Dorsal interossei [80]	Lateral plantar (tibial)	S1-2
• Tibialis posterior [76]	Tibial	L5-S1
• Flexor digitorum brevis [74]	Tibial	L4-S1
• Gastrocnemius [72]	Tibial	L5-S2
• Soleus [73]	Tibial	L5-S2
• Flexor hallucis longus [75]	Tibial	L5-S2
• Peroneus longus/brevis [71]	Superficial peroneal	L4-S1
• Tibialis anterior [66]	Deep peroneal	L4-S1
• Extensor hallucis longus [68]	Deep peroneal	L4-S1

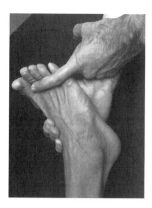

MUSCLE TESTING INSTRUCTIONS

Patient
Sitting or supine, the patient extends the toes.

Tester
The tester stabilizes the metatarsals while keeping the foot in slight plantar flexion. Resistance is generated against the proximal phalanges of toes 2 to 5.

Test
"Push your toes to your nose."

Pitfalls
A common mistake is to test ankle dorsiflexion instead of toe dorsiflexion.

CLINICAL PEARLS

1. The extensor digitorum longus [67] and the extensor digitorum brevis [70] tendons form conjoint tendons in toes 2 to 4 and thus both extend all these three toe joints. Toe 5 (the small toe) has no tendon from the extensor digitorum brevis [70] and can be used to detect extensor digitorum longus [67] weakness by assessing toe 5 metatarsophalangeal movement.

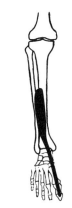

68. EXTENSOR HALLUCIS LONGUS

Origin
- Anterior middle third of the fibula

Insertion
- Distal phalanx of the great toe

Roots L5-S1

Nerve Deep peroneal

Open Chain Actions

SOLO ACTION
- Extension of the great toe (metatarsophalangeal and interphalangeal joints)

COMBINED ACTION
- Weak dorsiflexion of the ankle

Closed Chain Action Tilts the leg forward when the foot is fixed and flexes the knee

Synergists

Muscle	Nerve	Root
• Extensor digitorum brevis [70]	Deep peroneal	L5-S1
• Tibialis anterior [66]	Deep peroneal	L4-S1
• Extensor digitorum longus [67]	Deep peroneal	L4-S1
• Peroneus tertius [69]	Deep peroneal	L4-S1

Antagonists

Muscle	Nerve	Root
• Flexor hallucis longus [75]	Tibial	L5-S2
• Gastrocnemius [72]	Tibial	L5-S2
• Soleus [73]	Tibial	L5-S2
• Tibialis posterior [76]	Tibial	L5-S1
• Flexor digitorum longus [74]	Tibial	L5-S1
• Flexor hallucis longus [75]	Tibial	L5-S2
• Peroneus longus and brevis [71]	Superficial peroneal	L4-S1
• Abductor hallucis [77]	Medial plantar (tibial)	S1-2

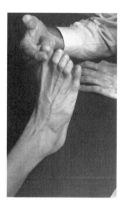

MUSCLE TESTING INSTRUCTIONS

Patient

In the neutral ankle position, the patient extends the interphalangeal and metatarsophalangeal joints of the great toe.

Tester

The tester generates pressure on the distal phalanx in a plantarflexion vector.

Test

"Bring your toe up toward your nose."

Pitfalls

Gout or bunions may cause a painful test.

CLINICAL PEARLS

1. The extensor hallucis longus [68] is a much more powerful muscle than the extensor hallucis brevis (medial slip of extensor digitorum brevis [70]).
2. The extensor hallucis longus [68] is the only muscle able to extend the interphalangeal joint of the great toe.
3. In clinical practice, the extensor hallucis longus [68] is commonly tested when suspecting an L5 radiculopathy.
4. The extensor hallucis longus [68] can dorsiflex the ankle (weakly).

69. PERONEUS TERTIUS

Origin
- Distal third of the fibula
- Interosseus membrane

Insertion
- Base of the fifth metatarsal (dorsal aspect)

Roots L4-S1

Nerve Deep peroneal

Open Chain Actions
SOLO ACTION
- Ankle dorsiflexion
- Foot eversion

COMBINED ACTION
- Foot eversion when balanced by the plantarflexors

Closed Chain Action Pulls the leg forward and laterally when the foot is fixed

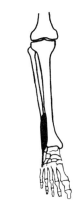

Synergists

Muscle	Nerve	Root
• Extensor digitorum longus [67]	Deep peroneal	L4-S1
• Extensor hallucis longus [68]	Deep peroneal	L5-S1
• Tibialis anterior [66]	Deep peroneal	L4-S1
• Peroneus longus and brevis [71]	Superficial peroneal	L4-S1

Antagonists

Muscle	Nerve	Root
• Flexor digitorum longus [74]	Tibial	L5-S1
• Tibialis posterior [76]	Tibial	L5-S1
• Gastrocnemius [72]	Tibial	L5-S2
• Soleus [73]	Tibial	L5-S2
• Flexor hallucis longus [75]	Tibial	L5-S2
• Peroneus longus and brevis [71]	Superficial peroneal	L4-S1
• Tibialis anterior [66]	Deep peroneal	L4-S1
• Extensor hallucis longus [68]	Deep peroneal	L5-S1

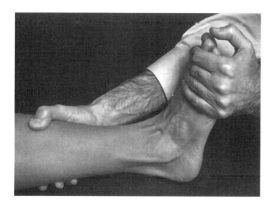

MUSCLE TESTING INSTRUCTIONS

Patient

Sitting or supine, the patient dorsiflexes and everts the foot.

Tester

The tester generates pressure along the dorsal and lateral aspects of the foot in a plan-tarflexion and inversion vector while stabilizing the distal leg with other hand.

Test

"Push your foot outward against my hand."

Pitfalls

This is a very small, weak muscle that is easily dominated by strong synergists. Thus, it is difficult to truly isolate.

CLINICAL PEARLS

1. The peroneus tertius [69] runs *anterior* to the ankle joint and is therefore an ankle *dorsiflexor.* The other peroneii tendons run behind the lateral malleolus, and thus plantarflex the ankle. All evert.

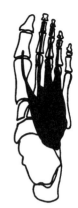

70. EXTENSOR DIGITORUM BREVIS

Origin
- Superior lateral aspect of the calcaneus

Insertion
- Base of the proximal phalanges of toes 1-4

Roots L5-S1

Nerve Deep peroneal

Open Chain Actions
SOLO ACTION
- Extends the metatarsophalangeal joints of toes 1 to 4 (not toe 5)

Copyright © 1997, McGraw-Hill.

COMBINED ACTION
- Extends the toes along with the extensor digitorum longus [67] and the extensor hallucis longus [68]

Closed Chain Action N/A

Synergists

Muscle	Nerve	Root
• Extensor hallucis longus [68]	Deep peroneal	L5-S1
• Extensor digitorum longus [67]	Deep peroneal	L4-S1

Antagonists

Muscle	Nerve	Root
• Flexor digitorum longus [74]	Tibial	L5-S1
• Flexor hallucis longus [75]	Tibial	L5-S2
• Abductor hallucis [77]	Medial plantar (tibial)	S1-S2
• Lumbricales [78]	Medial and lateral plantar (tibial)	L5-S2
• Plantar interossei [79]	Lateral plantar (tibial)	S1-2
• Dorsal interossei [80]	Lateral plantar (tibial)	S1-2

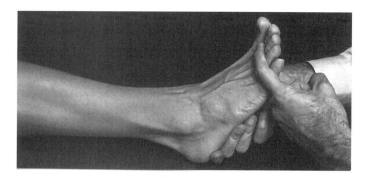

MUSCLE TESTING INSTRUCTIONS

Patient
Sitting or supine, the patient extends the toes

Tester
The tester stabilizes the metatarsals while keeping the foot in slight plantar flexion. Resistance is generated to the proximal phalanges of toes 2 to 5 in the flexion vector. The tester should observe or palpate the bulge of this muscle on the lateral aspect of the foot.

Test
"Point your toes to your nose."

Pitfalls
Ankle weakness can be mistaken for toe dorsiflexion weakness.

CLINICAL PEARLS

1. Toe 5 has no tendon from the extensor digitorum brevis [70] and can be used to detect extensor digitorum longus [67] weakness by assessing toe 5 metatarsophalangeal movement. The extensor digitorum longus [67] and extensor digitorum brevis [70] tendons form conjoint tendons in toes 2 to 4 by inserting into the middle and distal phalanges.

2. Some authors consider the extensor hallucis brevis (a muscle otherwise not discussed in this book) to really be a part of the extensor digitorum brevis [70].

71. PERONEUS LONGUS AND BREVIS

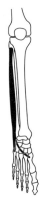

Origin
- Longus
  - Lateral condyle of the tibia
  - Proximal two-thirds of the fibula
  - Intermuscular septum
- Brevis
  - Distal two-thirds of the fibula
  - Intermuscular septum

Insertion
- Longus
  - Base of the first metatarsal
  - Medial cuneiform bone
- Brevis
  - Tuberosity on the base of the fifth metatarsal

Roots L4-S1

Nerve Superficial peroneal

Open Chain Actions
SOLO ACTION
- Ankle plantarflexion
- Foot eversion
- First metatarsal depression (longus)

COMBINED ACTION
- Plantarflexion when balanced by the inverters

Closed Chain Action Pulls the leg laterally when the foot is fixed

Synergists

Muscle	Nerve	Root
• Peroneus tertius [69]	Deep peroneal	L4-S1
• Flexor digitorum longus [74]	Tibial	L5-S1
• Tibialis posterior [76]	Tibial	L5-S1
• Flexor hallucis longus [75]	Tibial	L5-S2
• Gastrocnemius [72]	Tibial	L5-S2
• Soleus [73]	Tibial	L5-S2
• Extensor digitorum longus [67]	Deep peroneal	L4-S1

Antagonists

Muscle	Nerve	Root
• Tibialis anterior [66]	Deep peroneal	L4-S1
• Tibialis posterior [76]	Tibial	L5-S1
• Flexor digitorum longus [74]	Tibial	L5-S1
• Flexor hallucis longus [75]	Tibial	L5-S2
• Extensor hallucis longus [68]	Deep peroneal	L5-S1
• Extensor digitorum longus [67]	Deep peroneal	L4-S1
• Peroneus tertius [69]	Deep peroneal	L4-S1
• Gastrocnemius [72]	Tibial	L5-S2
• Soleus [73]	Tibial	L5-S2

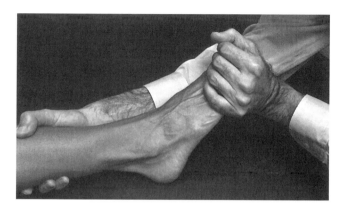

MUSCLE TESTING INSTRUCTIONS

Patient

Sitting or supine, the patient plantarflexes and everts the foot.

Tester

The tester stabilizes the distal leg and then generates a vector of inversion and dorsiflexion on the lateral aspect of the foot.

Test

"Push out and downward with your foot."

Pitfalls

It is difficult to isolate the strength of the peroneus longus [71] from that of the peroneus brevis [71].

CLINICAL PEARLS

1. The peroneus longus [71] wraps around the lateral foot and crosses under the metatarsals to insert into the first metatarsal. Look for first ray depression in order to assess activity and strength. Look at your own foot to understand the direction of pull.
2. The peroneus longus [71] lies in the proximal two-thirds of the leg. The peroneus brevis [71] lies in the distal two-thirds of the leg. The middle two-thirds of the leg, thus, has the two muscles overlapping. This anatomic fact should be remembered when palpating for muscle contraction.
3. The peroneus longus [71] and peroneus brevis [71] are the only muscles innervated by the superficial peroneal nerve.

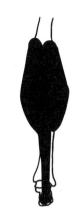

72. GASTROCNEMIUS

Origin
- Medial condyle of the femur
- Lateral condyle of the femur

Insertion
- The superior medial portion of the calcaneal tuberosity on the posterior calcaneus

Roots L5-S2

Nerve Tibial

Open Chain Actions
SOLO ACTION
- Ankle plantarflexion
- Knee flexion
- Mild ankle inversion

COMBINED ACTION
- Ankle plantarflexion
- Knee flexion
- Ankle inversion

Closed Chain Action Knee extension in stance

Synergists

Muscle	Nerve	Root
• Flexor digitorum longus [74]	Tibial	L5-S1
• Tibialis posterior [76]	Tibial	L5-S1
• Flexor hallucis longus [75]	Tibial	L5-S2
• Peroneus longus and brevis [71]	Superficial peroneal	L4-S1
• Soleus [73]	Tibial	L5-S2
• Semitendinosus/semimembranosus [64]	Tibial division of sciatic	L5-S2
• Biceps femoris [63]	Tibial, peroneal divisions of sciatic	L5-S2
• Gracilis [59]	Obturator	L2-4
• Sartorius [61]	Femoral	L2-4
• Tensor fascia lata [55]	Superior gluteal	L4-S1
• Popliteus [65]	Tibial	L4-S1
• Tibial anterior [66]	Deep peroneal	L4-S1
• Extensor hallucis longus [68]	Deep peroneal	L5-S1

Antagonists

Muscle	Nerve	Root
• Extensor digitorum longus [67]	Deep peroneal	L4-S1
• Extensor hallucis longus [68]	Deep peroneal	L5-S1
• Tibialis anterior [66]	Deep peroneal	L4-S1
• Peroneus tertius [69]	Deep peroneal	L4-S1
• Quadriceps [62]	Femoral	L2-4
• Peroneus longus and brevis [71]	Superficial peroneal	L4-S1

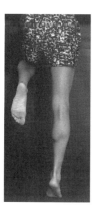

MUSCLE TESTING INSTRUCTIONS

Patient

Standing and holding on to something for balance, the patient pushes the body upward to rock onto the metatarsal heads. One can also assess, less objectively, by having the patient "Walk on the toes."

Tester

The tester stands beside the patient to ensure patient safety. The patient should be able to do ten unipedal toe raises. The tester should count and look for fatigue.

Test

"Rise up on your toes ten times on each foot."

Pitfalls

This is a very strong muscle; therefore, it is difficult to discern subtle weakness. This muscle should be tested in standing to fully assess the strength at grades 3 or better. One cannot grade the strength as "normal" if the tester is unable to "break" the strength of the muscle when patient is supine.

CLINICAL PEARLS

1. The gastrocnemius [72] crosses both the knee and the ankle joints. It is, therefore, able to act at both joints. This anatomic fact puts it at higher risk for shortening and contracture development.
2. Gastrocnemius [72] contracture is best assessed by the degree of passive ankle dorsiflexion attained with the knee fully flexed compared with the knee fully extended. The gastrocnemius [72] is most stretched when the knee is fully extended and the ankle fully dorsiflexed.
3. The gastrocnemius [72] is best stretched with full knee extension. The soleus [73] is best stretched with the knee flexed to slacken the gastrocnemius [72].
4. The gastrocnemius [72] is a two-joint muscle.

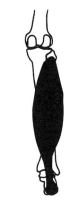

73. SOLEUS

Origin
- Posterior proximal one-third of the fibula
- Middle third of the tibia

Insertion
- Conjoins with the gastrocnemius [72] tendon to form the Achilles tendon inserting into the posterior calcaneus

Roots L5-S2

Nerve Tibial

Open Chain Actions
SOLO ACTION
- Ankle plantarflexion

COMBINED ACTION
- Ankle plantarflexion with gastrocnemius [72]
- Ankle inversion via the Achilles tendon

Closed Chain Action Pulls the leg posteriorly causing knee extension when the foot is fixed.

Synergists

Muscle	Nerve	Root
• Flexor digitorum longus [74]	Tibial	L5-S1
• Tibialis posterior [76]	Tibial	L5-S1
• Flexor hallucis longus [75]	Tibial	L5-S2
• Peroneus longus and brevis [71]	Superficial peroneal	L4-S1
• Gastrocnemius [72]	Tibial	L5-S2
• Tibialis anterior [66]	Deep peroneal	L4-S1
• Extensor hallucis longus [68]	Deep peroneal	L5-S1

Antagonists

Muscle	Nerve	Root
• Extensor digitorum longus [67]	Deep peroneal	L4-S1
• Extensor hallucis longus [68]	Deep peroneal	L5-S1
• Tibialis anterior [66]	Deep peroneal	L4-S1
• Peroneus tertius [69]	Deep peroneal	L4-S1
• Peroneus longus and brevis [71]	Superficial peroneal	L4-S1

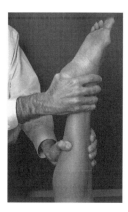

MUSCLE TESTING INSTRUCTIONS

Patient

Prone, the patient flexes the knee to 90 degrees.

Tester

The tester stabilizes the distal leg by holding the proximal ankle. The patient plantarflexes the ankle without inversion or eversion of the foot. The tester generates a dorsiflexion vector to assess the strength by pulling on the posterior calcaneus (significant weakness present) or with using the foot for leverage.

Test

"Point your foot toward the ceiling."

Pitfall

It is difficult to assess slight weakness (see gastrocnemius [72]).

CLINICAL PEARLS

1. Inversion during the described test suggests substitution by the tibialis posterior. Eversion suggests substitution by the peroneii.
2. The knee must be flexed to 90 degrees or more to "take out" the pull of the gastrocnemius [72].
3. Ankle plantarflexion contractures are almost always due to the gastrocnemius [72] shortening as it crosses two joints. The soleus [73] crosses only the ankle joint.

74. FLEXOR DIGITORUM LONGUS

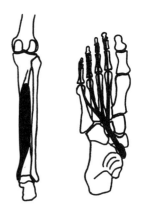

Origin
- Posterior aspect of the tibia

Insertion
- Distal phalanges of toes 2 to 5

Roots L5-S1

Nerve Tibial

Open Chain Actions
SOLO ACTION
- Toe flexion (toes 2 to 5)
- Ankle plantarflexion

COMBINED ACTION
- Toe flexion
- Ankle plantarflexion
- Ankle inversion

Closed Chain Action Extends the knee when the foot is fixed

Synergists

Muscle	Nerve	Root
• Lumbricales [78]	Medial and lateral plantar (tibial)	L5-S2
• Plantar interossei [79]	Lateral plantar (tibial)	S1-S2
• Dorsal interossei [80]	Lateral plantar (tibial)	S1-S2
• Tibialis posterior [76]	Tibial	L5-S1
• Flexor hallucis longus [75]	Tibial	L5-S2
• Peroneus longus and brevis [71]	Superficial peroneal	L4-S1
• Gastrocnemius [72]	Tibial	L5-S2
• Soleus [73]	Tibial	L5-S2
• Tibialis anterior [66]	Deep peroneal	L4-S1
• Extensor hallucis longus [68]	Deep peroneal	L5-S1

Antagonists

Muscle	Nerve	Root
• Extensor digitorum longus [67]	Deep peroneal	L4-S1
• Extensor hallucis longus [68]	Deep peroneal	L5-S1
• Extensor digitorum brevis [70]	Deep peroneal	L5-S1
• Tibialis anterior [66]	Deep peroneal	L4-S1
• Peroneus tertius [69]	Deep peroneal	L4-S1
• Peroneus longus and brevis [71]	Superficial peroneal	L4-S1

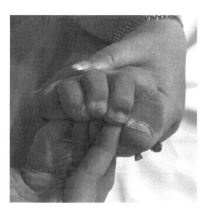

MUSCLE TESTING INSTRUCTIONS

Patient
Supine or sitting, the patient flexes the toes.

Tester
The tester generates an extension vector to the toes while stabilizing the mid-foot with the other hand.

Test
"Curl your toes down."

Pitfalls
N/A

CLINICAL PEARLS

1. Weakness can cause hyperextension of toes 2 to 5 and foot hyperpronation.
2. Even in complete paralysis of this muscle, the examiner might observe a flexion movement of the toes after active toe extension. This passive flexion of the toes is secondary to connective tissue recoil and must not be confused with true active toe flexion. Try passively flexing the toes slightly and then look for toe flexion movement.
3. It is difficult to distinguish the flexor digitorum brevis (otherwise not discussed in this book) from testing of the flexor digitorum longus [74].

75. FLEXOR HALLUCIS LONGUS

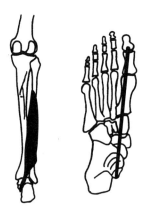

Origin
* Distal two-thirds of the fibula

Insertion
* Distal phalanx of the great toe

Roots L5-S2

Nerve Tibial

Open Chain Actions
SOLO ACTION
* Great toe flexion
* Ankle plantarflexion
* Foot inversion

COMBINED ACTION
* Great toe flexion
* Ankle plantarflexion
* Foot inversion

Closed Chain Action Pulls the foot forward and assists in knee extension when the foot is fixed

Synergists

Muscle	Nerve	Root
• Abductor hallucis [77]	Medial plantar	S1-S2
• Flexor digitorum longus [74]	Tibial	L5-S1
• Tibialis posterior [76]	Tibial	L5-S1
• Peroneus longus and brevis [71]	Superficial peroneal	L4-S1
• Gastrocnemius [72]	Tibial	L5-S1
• Soleus [73]	Tibial	L5-S2
• Tibialis anterior [66]	Deep peroneal	L4-S1
• Extensor hallucis longus [68]	Deep peroneal	L5-S1

Antagonists

Muscle	Nerve	Root
• Extensor hallucis longus [68]	Deep peroneal	L5-S1
• Extensor digitorum brevis [70]	Deep peroneal	L5-S1
• Extensor digitorum longus [67]	Deep peroneal	L4-S1
• Tibialis anterior [66]	Deep peroneal	L4-S1
• Peroneus tertius [69]	Deep peroneal	L4-S1
• Peroneus longus and brevis [71]	Superficial peroneal	L4-S1

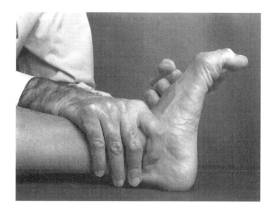

MUSCLE TESTING INSTRUCTIONS

Patient
Supine or sitting, the patient flexes the great toe.

Tester
The tester generates an extension vector to the great toe while stabilizing the metatarsals with other hand.

Test
"Curl your big toe down."

Pitfalls
If the ankle is not kept in a neutral position between dorsiflexion and plantarflexion, the big toe might passively flex secondary to a tight tendon.

CLINICAL PEARLS

1. It may be difficult for the patient to isolate the motion of this toe from the other toes.

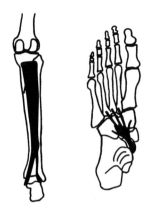

76. TIBIALIS POSTERIOR

Origin
- Proximal two-thirds of the tibia
- Proximal two-thirds of the fibula
- Interosseus membrane

Insertion
- Navicular
- With extensions to the cuneiforms
- With extensions to the cuboid
- With extensions to the 2 to 4 metatarsals

Roots L5-S1

Nerve Tibial

Open Chain Actions
SOLO ACTION
- Foot inversion
- Ankle plantarflexion

COMBINED ACTION
- Foot inversion
- Ankle plantarflexion

Closed Chain Action Knee extension when the foot is fixed

Synergists

Muscle	Nerve	Root
• Flexor digitorum longus [74]	Tibial	L5-S1
• Flexor hallucis longus [75]	Tibial	L5-S2
• Peroneus longus and brevis [71]	Superficial peroneal	L4-S1
• Gastrocnemius [72]	Tibial	L5-S2
• Soleus [73]	Tibial	L5-S2
• Tibialis anterior [66]	Deep peroneal	L4-S1
• Extensor hallucis longus [68]	Deep peroneal	L5-S1

Antagonists

Muscle	Nerve	Root
• Peroneus longus and brevis [71]	Superficial peroneal	L4-S1
• Peroneus tertius [69]	Deep peroneal	L4-S1
• Extensor digitorum longus [67]	Deep peroneal	L4-S1
• Extensor hallucis longus [68]	Deep peroneal	L5-S1
• Tibialis anterior [66]	Deep peroneal	L4-S1

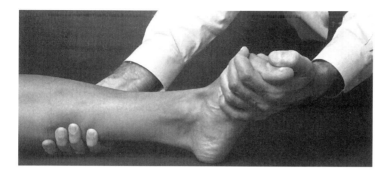

MUSCLE TESTING INSTRUCTIONS

Patient

Supine or sitting, the patient plantarflexes and inverts the foot and ankle.

Tester

The tester is sitting or standing beside the patient. The tester generates an eversion and dorsiflexion vector to the foot and ankle.

Test

"Push your foot down and inward."

Pitfalls

The flexor hallucis longus [75] and flexor digitorum longus [74] can substitute for this muscle's actions. Watch for strong flexion by these muscles.

CLINICAL PEARLS

1. The tibialis posterior [76] is a major contributor to the longitudinal foot arch. A tear or rupture of this muscle can cause significant foot pronation.
2. The tibialis posterior [76] is another culprit in equinovarus contracture of the ankle, along with the gastrocnemius [72].
3. In electrodiagnostic studies, the tibialis posterior [76] has been found to be a very pure L5-innervated muscle.

77. ABDUCTOR HALLUCIS

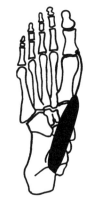

Origin
- Medial calcaneus
- Flexor retinaculum
- Plantar aponeurosis

Insertion
- Proximal phalanx of the great toe

Roots S1-2

Nerve Medial plantar

Open Chain Actions
SOLO ACTION
- Abducts the great toe
- Stabilizes the first metatarsal

COMBINED ACTION
- Flexes the metatarsophalangeal joint of the great toe along with the toe flexors
- Adducts the forefoot

Closed Chain Action N/A

Synergists

Muscle	Nerve	Root
• Flexor hallucis longus [75]	Tibial	L5-S2

Antagonists

Muscle	Nerve	Root
• Adductor hallucis	Lateral plantar	S1-2
• Extensor hallucis longus [68]	Deep peroneal	L5-S1
• Extensor digitorum brevis [70]	Deep peroneal	L5-S1

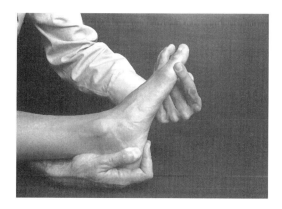

MUSCLE TESTING INSTRUCTIONS

Patient
Supine or sitting, the patient attempts to abduct the great toe.

Tester
The tester is sitting or standing beside the patient. The tester generates an adduction vector to the great toe while palpating the muscle belly just inferior and posterior to the navicular.

Test
"Push against my finger with your big toe."

Pitfalls
It is often difficult to voluntarily contract this muscle.

CLINICAL PEARLS

1. Abductor hallucis [77] weakness can contribute to foot deformities (forefoot valgus, hallux valgus, and medial migration of the navicular).
2. A common muscle tested in electrodiagnostic studies of the lower extremities.

78. LUMBRICALES

Origin
- Flexor digitorum longus [74] tendons (toes 2 to 5)

Insertion
- Toe extensor tendons

Roots
- L5-S1 (lumbricale 1)
- S1-2 (lumbricales 2 to 4)

Nerve
- Medial plantar (lumbricale 1)
- Lateral plantar (lumbricales 2 to 4)

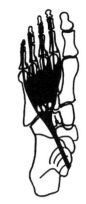

Open Chain Actions
SOLO ACTION
- Flexion of the metatarsophalangeal joints 2 to 4

COMBINED ACTION
- Flexion of the metatarsophalangeal joints 2 to 4
- Extension of the interphalangeal joints
- Stabilizes the forefoot

Closed Chain Action N/A

Synergists

Muscle	Nerve	Root
• Flexor digitorum longus [74]	Tibial	L5-S1

Antagonists

Muscle	Nerve	Root
• Extensor digitorum longus [67]	Deep peroneal	L4-S1
• Extensor digitorum brevis [70]	Deep peroneal	L5-S1

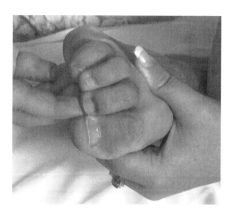

MUSCLE TESTING INSTRUCTIONS

Patient
Supine or sitting, the patient flexes the metatarsophalangeal joints of the feet.

Tester
The tester is sitting or standing beside the patient. The tester generates an extension vector under the metatarsophalangeal joints of toes 2 to 4.

Test
"Curl your toes down."

Pitfalls
N/A

CLINICAL PEARLS

1. Lumbricale [78] atrophy and weakness are major contributors to hammer toes and loss of the transverse foot arch.

79. PLANTAR INTEROSSEI

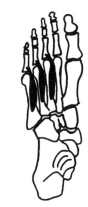

Origin
- Bases and the medial aspects of metatarsals 3 to 5

Insertion
- Medial aspects of the proximal phalanges of the same digits
- Dorsal aponeuroses of the extensor digitorum longus [67]

Roots S1-2

Nerve Lateral plantar

Open Chain Actions
SOLO ACTION
- Adducts digits 2 to 5

COMBINED ACTION
- Metatarsophalangeal joint flexion in digits 3 to 5 with the other toe flexors
- Weakly extends the interphalangeal joint of digits 3 to 5
- Stabilizes the forefoot

Closed Chain Action N/A

Synergists

Muscle	Nerve	Root
• Flexor digitorum longus [74]	Tibial	L5-S1
• Flexor hallucis longus [75]	Tibial	L5-S2
• Lumbricales (2 to 4) [78]	Lateral plantar (tibial)	S1-2

Antagonists

Muscle	Nerve	Root
• Dorsal interossei [80]	Lateral plantar (tibial)	S1-2

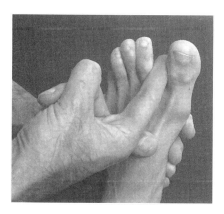

MUSCLE TESTING INSTRUCTIONS

Patient

Supine or sitting, the patient adducts the toes.

Tester

The tester is sitting or standing beside the patient. The tester stabilizes the metatarsophalangeal joints and puts a finger between each toe. The passive and active medial and lateral movement of the toes should be assessed.

Test

"Push your toes to the right and then left."

Pitfalls

N/A

CLINICAL PEARLS

1. A questionably useful muscle to manually test, but one should know its anatomy and be alert for contractures.

80. DORSAL INTEROSSEI

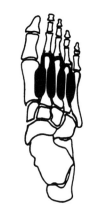

Origin
• Four, each from two heads of the adjacent metatarsals

Insertion
• Sides of the proximal phalanx (lateral side of digits 2 to 4; medial side of digit 2)

Roots S1-2

Nerve Lateral plantar

Open Chain Actions
SOLO ACTION
• Abducts digits 2 to 4

COMBINED ACTION
• Assists in flexion of the metatarsophalangeal joints of digits 2 to 4
• Weakly assists in extension of the interphalangeal joints of digits 2 to 4
• Stabilizes the forefoot

Closed Chain Action N/A

Synergists

Muscle	Nerve	Root
• Flexor digitorum longus [74]	Tibial	L5-S1
• Flexor hallucis longus [75]	Tibial	L5-S2
• Lumbricales (2 to 4) [78]	Lateral plantar (tibial)	S1-2

Antagonists

Muscle	Nerve	Root
• Plantar interossei [79]	Lateral plantar (tibial)	S1-2

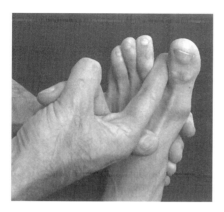

MUSCLE TESTING INSTRUCTIONS

Patient
Supine, sitting, or prone the patient abducts the toes

Tester
The tester is sitting or standing beside the patient. The tester stabilizes the metatarsophalangeal joints and puts a finger between each toe. The passive and active medial and lateral movements of the toes should be assessed.

Test
"Push your toes to the right and then left."

Pitfalls
N/A

CLINICAL PEARLS

1. A questionably useful muscle to manually test, but one should know its anatomy and be alert for contractures.

81. ABDUCTOR DIGITI MINIMI

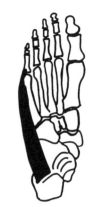

Origin
- Calcaneal tuberosity and its medial and lateral processes
- Adjacent fascia

Insertion
- Lateral side of the proximal fifth digit

Roots S1-2

Nerve Lateral plantar

Open Chain Actions
SOLO ACTION
- Abducts the fifth digit

COMBINED ACTION
- Assists in flexion of the interphalangeal joint of the fifth digit
- Stabilizes the forefoot

Copyright © 1997, McGraw-Hill.

Closed Chain Action N/A

Synergists

Muscle	Nerve	Root
• Flexor digitorum longus [74]	Tibial	L5-S1
• Lumbricales (fourth) [78]	Lateral plantar (tibial)	S1-2

Antagonists

Muscle	Nerve	Root
• Plantar interossei (fifth) [79]	Lateral plantar (tibial)	S1-2

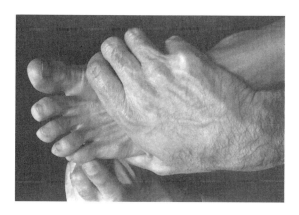

MUSCLE TESTING INSTRUCTIONS

Patient
Supine or sitting, the patient attempts to abduct the little toe.

Tester
The tester is sitting or standing beside the patient. While stabilizing the metatarsopha-langeal joint of the fifth digit, an adduction or medial vector is generated.

Test
"Push your little toe outward against my finger."

Pitfalls
This muscle is difficult for many people to isolate.

CLINICAL PEARLS

N/A

QUESTIONS

1. To which digits does the extensor digitorum longus [67] insert? Extensor digitorum brevis [70]?
2. Where does the tibialis anterior [66] insert? Why might that be important in partial foot amputations?
3. Describe the origin and insertion of the tibialis posterior [76]. What role might it play in foot architecture?
4. Name the nerve and root level innervation of the tibialis posterior [76] and explain how one might use this information for discerning a peroneal neuropathy versus an L5 radiculopathy.
5. Describe the origin, course, and insertion of the peroneus longus and peroneus brevis [71].
6. How can you differentiate the soleus [73] from gastrocnemius [72] tightness? Which one usually causes contractures at the ankle and why?
7. Name the L4 innervated muscles below the knee.
8. Name the L5 innervated muscles below the ankle.
9. Name muscles at or below the knee that can assist with knee extension. Why?
10. Name the tendons palpated on the anterior ankle when moving your fingers from the medial malleolus to the lateral maleolus.

CHAPTER 7

TRUNK AND PARASPINALS

Scott Nadler and Todd Stitik

T6-T12
- **82.** Rectus abdominis
- **83.** External abdominal oblique
- **84.** Internal abdominal oblique
- **85.** Quadratus lumborum

DORSAL ROOTS
- **86.** Iliocostalis cervicis, thoracis, and lumborum
- **87.** Longissimus capitis, cervicis, and thoracis
- **88.** Spinalis capitis, cervicis, and throacis
- **89.** Semispinalis capitis and cervicis
- **90.** Multifidus
- **91.** Rotatores

MUSCLES OMITTED
Intertransverseri
Semispinalis thoracis

82. RECTUS ABDOMINIS

Origin
- Pubic crest

Insertion
- Xyphoid process
- Costal cartilages of ribs 5, 6, and 7

Roots T5-12 (ventral rami)

Trunk N/A

Cord N/A

Nerve 7th-11th Intercostal nerves

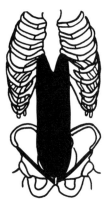

Muscle Actions
- Compresses the abdominopelvic cavity
- Flexes the vertebral column by approximating the thorax and pelvis anteriorly
- Assists the neck flexors in raising the head from a supine position by fixing the thorax

Synergists

Muscle	Nerve	Root
• Internal abdominal oblique [84]	Intercostals, iliohypogastric, ilioinguinal	T5-L1
• External abdominal oblique [83]	Intercostals, iliohypogastric, ilioinguinal	T5-L1
• Transversus abdominis	Intercostals, iliohypogastric, ilioinguinal	T6-12

Antagonists

Muscle	Nerve	Root
• Iliocostalis thoracis [86]	Direct branches of spinal nerves	Thoracic roots
• Iliocostalis lumborum [86]	Direct branches of spinal nerves	Lumbar roots
• Interspinales	Direct branches of spinal nerves	Thoracolumbar roots
• Longissimus thoracis [87]	Direct branches of spinal nerves	Thoracic roots
• Spinalis thoracis [88]	Direct branches of spinal nerves	Thoracic roots

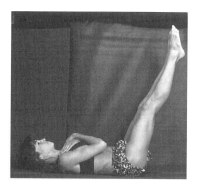 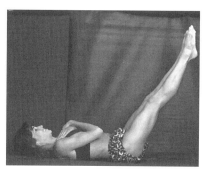

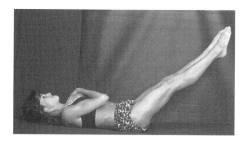 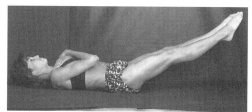

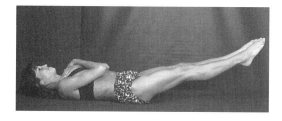 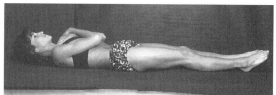

MUSCLE TESTING INSTRUCTIONS

A. GRADING LOWER ABDOMINAL STRENTGH: LEG-LOWERING TEST

It is not possible to solely isolate out the action of the rectus abdominis [82] muscle since the external abdominal oblique [83] also participates in this test.

Patient

Supine on a firm surface with the forearms folded across the chest.

Tester

- The tester may assist the patient in positioning the legs (knees straight) to a vertical (90 degrees) position.
- The tester watches to ensure that the patient is not assisting himself/herself by using the elbows against the table or grabbing onto the sides of the table.
- The tester notes the angle between the extended legs and the table at the moment the pelvis starts to tilt anteriorly and the low back arches from the table.
- The tester uses this angle to assign a muscle strength grade based on the chart below:

Angle (Degrees)	Muscle Grade (Verbal)	Muscle Grade (Numerical)
90	Poor	2
75	Fair	3
60	Fair (+)	3+
45	Good (−)	4−
30	Good	4
15	Good (+)	4+
0	Normal	5

Test

"Flatten your low back against the table by contracting the abdominal muscles and hold your back flat while slowly lowering the legs until they touch the table."

Pitfalls

- Hamstring tightness may interfere with achieving a full vertical starting position.
- Helping the patient stabilize the trunk defeats the purpose of the test.
- If the forearms are not folded across the chest, the elbows could potentially be resting on the table for support or the patient might grab onto the sides of the table for assistance.

Clinical Pearls

The following combinations of strength and weakness (in order of decreasing frequency) of the abdominal muscles as a whole are generally found:

- Upper abdominal muscles strong and lower abdominal muscles weak
- Upper abdominal muscles and lower abdominal muscles both weak
- Upper abdominal muscles and lower abdominal muscles both strong
- Lower abdominal muscles strong and upper abdominal muscles weak

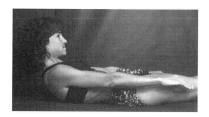 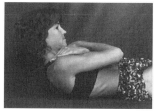 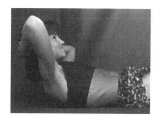

B. GRADING UPPER ABDOMINAL STRENGTH: CURLED TRUNK SIT-UPS

As is true for the leg-lowering test, it is not possible to solely isolate out the action of the rectus abdominis [82] muscle using this test. Both the external [83] and internal abdominal obliques [84] also participate.

Patient

Lies supine with the legs extended, clasps hands behind the head, slowly raises the head and shoulders from the supine position until the trunk curl is completed. Enters without hesitation into the hip flexion phase and stops when he/she reaches a full long-sit position.

Tester

The tester may hold the feet down but not until the patient enters the hip flexion phase of the movement. Observes the patient during both trunk curl phase (spine flexion) and sit-up (hip flexion) and grades the muscle strength as follows:

- *Fair:* With the arms extended forward, the patient can flex the vertebral column but cannot maintain flexion when attempting to enter the hip flexion phase.
- *Fair (+):* With the arms extended forward, the patient can flex the vertebral column and can maintain flexion when entering the hip flexion phase and coming to a seated position.
- *Good:* With the arms folded across the chest, the patient is able to flex the vertebral column and can maintain flexion when entering the hip flexion phase and coming to a seated position.
- *Normal:* With the hands clasped behind the head, the patient is able to flex the vertebral column and can maintain flexion when entering the hip flexion phase and coming to a seated position.

Test

"Do a sit-up while keeping your legs straight and hands behind your head. If you are unable to do this, then attempt it with the arms folded across the chest. If you are still unable to do this, then perform the test with your arms straight out in front of you."

Pitfalls

- Do not hold the patient's feet down during the trunk curl phase. Doing this allows the hip flexors to initiate trunk raising by flexing the pelvis on the thighs (i.e., the hip flexors are fixed and allow the patient to perform an arched back sit-up). Holding down the feet during the hip flexion phase is permissible. In fact, if the patient is unable to keep the heels in contact with the table, the lower abdominal muscles will also contribute to the test, and the movement will no longer isolate the upper abdominal muscles.

- Since the hip flexion phase provides strong resistance against the abdominal muscles (because the hip flexors pull strongly downward on the pelvis as the abdominals work to hold the pelvis in the direction of the posterior tilt), stopping the movement before entering the hip flexion phase will not allow muscle strength to be properly assessed.

- When the patient enters the hip flexion phase of the movement, the tester must make sure that the pelvis remains posteriorly tilted (low back flat), otherwise the hip flexors rather than the upper abdominal muscles will actually be completing the movement.

Clinical Pearls

1. Prior to doing the test, check the range of motion of the lumbosacral spine so as to avoid misinterpretation of motion restriction as weakness.

2. Prior to doing the test, perform the Thomas test to rule out hip flexor tightness since tight hip flexors can prevent posterior pelvic tilting that is needed to cause flattening of the lumbar spine. (The Thomas test is performed by having the supine patient individually flex each hip into the chest monitoring for elevation of the opposite hip from the table.) Tightness of the hip flexor is indicated by elevation of the opposite thigh off of the table. If the hip flexors are tight, place a rolled towel under the knees so as to passively flex the hips enough to allow the low back to flatten.

3. In order to grade the muscle strength, only one properly performed curled trunk sit-up needs to be done.

4. The rectus abdominis [82], the internal abdominal obliques [84], and the external abdominal obliques [83] contribute to this movement as follows:
   - Rectus abdominis [82]: depresses the chest and pulls the thorax toward the pelvis
   - Internal abdominal obliques [84]: flare out the rib cage
   - External abdominal obliques [83]: become active when the patient enters the hip flexion phase of the movement and acts to pull the rib cage inward again

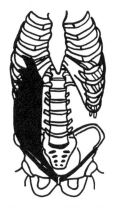

83. EXTERNAL ABDOMINAL OBLIQUE

Origin
- Lower border of the eight inferior ribs

Insertion
- Lower fibers insert into the anterior half of the outer lip of the crest of the ilium
- Middle and upper fibers insert in an aponeurosis that interlaces with the opposite side muscle forming the linea alba

Roots T5-L1

Trunk N/A

Cord N/A

Copyright © 1997, McGraw-Hill.

Nerve
- Intercostal nerves: T5-12
- Iliohypogastric: T12-L1
- Ilioinguinal: L1

Muscle Actions
- Trunk rotation to the opposite side
- Pelvic elevation
- Lateral flexion of the trunk
- Flexion of the vertebral column when firing bilaterally

Synergists

Muscle	Nerve	Root
• Rectus abdominis [82]	Intercostals	T5-12
• Internal abdominal obliques [84]	Intercostals, iliohypogastric, ilioinguinal	T5-L1
• Transversus abdominis	Intercostals, iliohypogastric, ilioinguinal	T6-12

Antagonists

Muscle	Nerve	Root
• Iliocostalis thoracis [86]	Direct branches of spinal nerves	Thoracic roots
• Iliocostalis lumborum [86]	Direct branches of spinal nerves	Lumbar roots
• Interspinalis	Direct branches of spinal nerves	Thoracolumbar roots
• Longissimus thoracis [87]	Direct branches of spinal nerves	Thoracic roots
• Spinalis thoracis [88]	Direct branches of spinal nerves	Thoracic roots
• Multifidus [90]	Direct branches of spinal nerves	Thoracolumbar roots

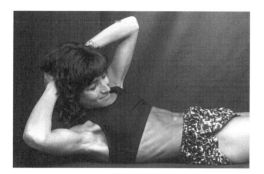

MUSCLE TESTING INSTRUCTIONS

Patient

Supine with the hands behind the neck

Tester

The tester stabilizes the lower limbs.

- *Good:* Denoted by full elevation of the rotating shoulder and only partial elevation of the opposite shoulder.
- *Fair:* Denoted by only elevation of the rotating shoulder.

Test

"Do a sit-up and twist your body to the side."

Pitfalls

If hip the flexors are weak, the pelvis must be stabilized.

CLINICAL PEARLS

1. Rotation of the trunk is accomplished via ipsilateral external abdominal oblique [83] and contralateral internal abdominal oblique [84].
2. Unilateral weakness of lateral fibers of internal [84]/external abdominal obliques [83] leads to C-curve convex to the side of weakness (lateral shift of pelvis).
3. Moderate weakness of the external abdominal oblique [83] decreases respiratory efficiency and support of the abdominal viscera.
4. Bilateral weakness of the external abdominal oblique [83] leads to decreased ability to flex the vertebral column and tilt the pelvis posteriorly.

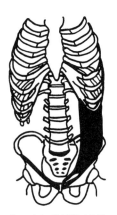

84. INTERNAL ABDOMINAL OBLIQUE

Origin
- Inguinal ligament
- Iliac crest
- Lumbodorsal fascia

Insertion
- Pubic crest
- Lower four ribs
- Linea alba (an aponeurosis formed with the muscles on the opposite side)

Roots T5-L1

Trunk N/A

Cord N/A

Nerve
- Intercostal nerves: T5-12
- Iliohypogastric: T12-L1
- Ilioinguinal: L1

Muscle Actions
- Trunk rotation
- Pelvic elevation
- Lateral flexion of the trunk
- Flexion of the vertebral column when the muscle is activated bilaterally

Synergists

Muscle	Nerve	Root
• Rectus abdominis [82]	Intercostals	T5-12
• External abdominal obliques [83]	Intercostals, iliohypogastric, ilioinguinal	T5-12
• Transversus abdominis	Intercostals, iliohypogastric, ilioinguinal	T6-12

Antagonists Trunk extensors

Muscle	Nerve	Root
• Iliocostalis thoracis [86]	Direct branches of spinal nerves	Thoracic roots
• Iliocostalis lumborum [86]	Direct branches of spinal nerves	Lumbar roots
• Interspinales	Direct branches of spinal nerves	Thoracolumbar roots
• Longissimus thoracis [87]	Direct branches of spinal nerves	Thoracic roots
• Spinalis thoracis [88]	Direct branches of spinal nerves	Thoracic roots
• Multifidus [90]	Direct branches of spinal nerves	Thoracolumbar roots

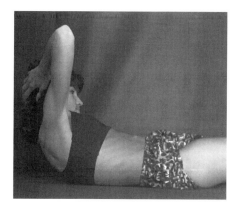

MUSCLE TESTING INSTRUCTIONS

Patient   Supine with the hands clasped behind the head.

Tester   The tester stabilizes the lower limbs.
- *Good:* Denoted by full elevation of the rotating shoulder and only partial elevation of the opposite shoulder.
- *Fair:* Denoted by only elevation of the rotating shoulder.

Test   "Do a sit-up and twist your body to the side."

Pitfalls   If the hip flexors are weak, the pelvis must be stabilized

CLINICAL PEARLS

1. Moderate or marked weakness of the internal [84] and external abdominal obliques [83] decreases respiratory efficiency and support of the abdominal viscera.
2. Weakness of an internal abdominal oblique [84] (along with weakness of an external abdominal oblique) can play a role in scoliosis as follows:
   - A weak left internal abdominal oblique and a weak right external abdominal oblique leads to a separation of the right costal margin from the left iliac crest, thus the thorax deviates toward the right and rotates posteriorly on the right. This promotes a right thoracic and left lumbar scoliosis. The opposite effect would occur with a weak right internal abdominal oblique and a weak left external abdominal oblique.
   - A weak ipsilateral internal abdominal oblique and external abdominal oblique leads to separation of the thorax and iliac crest laterally, resulting in a C-curve convex toward the weak side.
3. Bilateral shortness of the internal [84] and external [83] obliques causes anterior depression of the thorax leading to flexion of the vertebral column. Hence, kyphosis and a depressed chest will result.
4. It is not possible to completely isolate the actions of the internal abdominal oblique [84] muscles from those of the other abdominal muscles. The technique used in assessment of the external abdominal oblique [83] may be used to directly evaluate function of the obliques. Remember that rotation is accomplished via activation of the ipsilateral external abdominal oblique [83] and the contralateral internal abdominal oblique [84]. Performance of a curled trunk sit-up can assess its function indirectly.

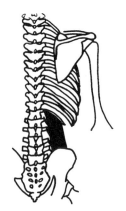

85. QUADRATUS LUMBORUM

Origin
- Iliolumbar ligament
- Crest of the ilium
- Occasionally, it also arises from the lower three lumbar transverse processes

Insertion
- Lower border of the 12th rib
- Transverse processes of the upper four lumbar vertebrae
- Lower margin of 12th rib.

Roots Ventral division of roots T12-L1

Trunk N/A

Cord N/A

Nerve N/A

Muscle Actions
- Elevation of the pelvis
- Pulls down the 12th rib acting as a muscle of inspiration to fix the origin of the diaphragm
- Extension of the trunk
- Flexion of the trunk (when bilateral quadratus lumborum [85] are activated)
- Lateral flexion of the trunk

Synergists

Muscle	Nerve	Root
• Iliocostalis lumborum [86]	Direct braches of spinal nerves	Lumbar roots
• External abdominal oblique [83]	Intercostals, iliohypogastric, ilioinguinal	T5-L1
• Gluteus medius [53]	Superior gluteal	L4-S1
• Gluteus minimus [54]	Superior gluteal	L4-S1
• Semispinalis [89]	Direct branches of spinal nerves	Lumbar roots
• Multifidi [90]	Direct branches of spinal nerves	Lumbar roots
• Rotatores [91]	Direct branches of spinal nerves	Lumbar roots

Antagonists

Muscle	Nerve	Root
• Contralateral quadratus lumborum [85]	Direct branch of spinal nerves	T12-L1
• Contralateral external abdominal oblique [83]	Intercostals, iliohypogastric, ilioinguinal	T5-L1
• Contralateral internal abdominal oblique [84]	Intercostals, iliohypogastric, ilioinguinal	T5-L1

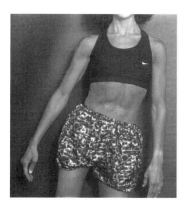

MUSCLE TESTING INSTRUCTIONS

Patient

Technique 1: The patient stands with the feet spread equidistant to pelvis.

Technique 2: The patient is supine with lumbar lordosis maintained.

Tester

Technique 1: The tester stands behind the patient supporting the upper trunk.

Technique 2: The tester provides resistance above the ankle joint.

Test

"Try to bring your ribs and hip together on one side."

Pitfalls

The patient may attempt to side bend the trunk toward the side instead of elevating the pelvis.

CLINICAL PEARLS

1. Evaluate both sides for any differences in ease of performing this test.
2. The quadratus lumborum [85] may be a key muscle in controlling lumbar facet motion. It should be assessed in all patients with subacute and chronic low back pain.
3. May be assessed with the patient in side-lying position with knee and hip flexed to 90 degrees. The tester stabilizes the trunk and asks the patient to elevate his/her feet toward the ceiling.
4. Trunk flexion is a combination of lateral tilting of the pelvis and hip adduction. Muscles involved include the lateral fibers of the internal [84]/external [83] obliques, quadratus lumborum [85], latissimus dorsi [7], and ipsilateral rectus abdominus [82].

86. ILIOCOSTALIS CERVICIS, THORACIS, AND LUMBORUM

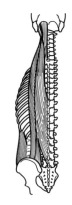

Origin
- Iliocostalis cervicis
  - Angles of the 3rd to 6th ribs
- Iliocostalis thoracis
  - Angles of lower 6 ribs
- Iliocostalis lumborum
  - Sacral crest
  - Spinous processes of T11-12 and lumbar vertebrae
  - Iliac crests
  - Supraspinous ligament

Insertion
- Iliocostalis cervicis
  - Transverse processes of the cervical vertebrae (C4-6)
- Iliocostalis thoracis
  - Transverse process of C7
  - Angles of the upper 6 ribs
- Iliocostalis lumborum
  - Angles of the lower 6 or 7 ribs

Roots Cervical, thoracic, and lumbar nerve roots

Trunk N/A

Cord N/A

Nerve Direct branches off of spinal nerve roots

Muscle Actions
- Extends the vertebral column
- Lateral flexion of the vertebral column to the same side
- Rotation to the same side

Synergists

Muscle	Nerve	Root
Interspinales	Direct branches of spinal nerves	C, T, L roots
Longissimus cervicis [87]	Direct branches of spinal nerves	Cervical roots
Longissimus thoracis [87]	Direct branches of spinal nerves	Thoracic roots
Multifidi [90]	Direct branches of spinal nerves	C, T, L roots
Quadratus lumborum [85]	Direct branches of spinal nerves	T12-L1
Rotatores [91]	Direct branches of spinal nerves	C, T, L roots
Semispinalis capitis [89]	Direct branches of spinal nerves	Cervical roots
Semispinalis cervicis [89]	Direct branches of spinal nerves	Cervical roots
Spinalis capitis [88]	Direct branches of spinal nerves	Cervical roots
Spinalis cervicis[88]	Direct branches of spinal nerves	Cervical roots
Spinalis thoracis [88]	Direct branches of spinal nerves	Thoracic roots

Antagonists

Muscle	Nerve	Root
• Rectus capitis anticus major	Direct branch of spinal nerve	C1-2
• Rectus capitis anticus minor	Direct branch of spinal nerve	C1-2
• Rectus capitis lateralis	Direct branch of spinal nerve	C1-2
• Longus colli	Direct branch of spinal nerve	C5-8
• Scalenus anticus [108]	Direct branch of spinal nerve	C3-8
• Scalenus medius [108]	Direct branch of spinal nerve	C3-8
• Sternocleidomastoid [107]	Spinal accessory nerve	C2-3
• Internal abdominals obliques [84]	Intercostals, iliohypogastric, ilioinguinal	T5-L1
• External abdominals obliques [83]	Intercostals, iliohypogastric, ilioinguinal	T5-L1
• Rectus abdominus [82]	Intercostals	T5-12

MUSCLE TESTING INSTRUCTIONS

See "Spine Extension Testing"

CLINICAL PEARLS

See "Spine Extension Testing"

87. LONGISSIMUS CAPITIS, CERVICIS, AND THORACIS

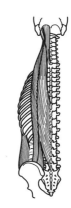

Origin
- Longissimus capitis and cervicis
  - Transverse processes of first 4 or 5 thoracic vertebrae
  - Articular processes of last 3 or 4 cervical vertebra
- Longissimus thoracis
  - Posterior surface of the lumbar transverse processes
  - Anterior layer of the thoracolumbar fascia

Insertion
- Longissimus capitis: posterior margin of the mastoid
- Longissimus cervicis: posterior tubercle of transverse processes of 2nd to 6th cervical vertebra.
- Longissimus thoracis: transverse processes of thoracic vertebra and into lower 9 or 10 ribs between the tubercle and rib angle

Roots Cervical and thoracic nerve roots

Trunk N/A

Cord N/A

Nerve N/A

Muscle Actions
- Extends the vertebral column
- Lateral flexion of the vertebral column
- Rotation to same side

Synergists

Muscle	Nerve	Root
• Interspinales	Direct branches of spinal nerves	C, T, L roots
• Iliocostalis cervicis [86]	Direct branches of spinal nerves	Cervical roots
• Iliocostalis thoracis [86]	Direct branches of spinal nerves	Thoracic roots
• Multifidi [90]	Direct branches of spinal nerves	C, T, L roots
• Rotatores [91]	Direct branches of spinal nerves	C, T, L roots
• Semispinalis capitis [89]	Direct branches of spinal nerves	Cervical roots
• Semispinalis cervicis [89]	Direct branches of spinal nerves	Cervical roots
• Spinalis capitis [88]	Direct branches of spinal nerves	Cervical roots
• Spinalis cervicis [88]	Direct branches of spinal nerves	Cervical roots
• Spinalis thoracis [88]	Direct branches of spinal nerves	Thoracic roots

Antagonists

Muscle	Nerve	Root
• Rectus capitis anticus major	Direct branch of spinal nerve	C1-2
• Rectus capitis anticus minor	Direct branch of spinal nerve	C1-2
• Rectus capitis lateralis	Direct branch of spinal nerve	C1-2
• Longus colli	Direct branch of spinal nerve	C5-8
• Scalenus anticus [108]	Direct branch of spinal nerve	C3-C8
• Scalenus medius [108]	Direct branch of spinal nerve	C3-C8
• Sternocleidomastoid [107]	Spinal accessory nerve	C2-3
• Internal abdominal obliques [84]	Intercostals, iliohypogastric, ilioinguinal	T5-L1
• External abdominal obliques [83]	Intercostals, iliohypogastric, ilioinguinal	T5-L1
• Rectus abdominus [82]	Intercostals	T5-12

MUSCLE TESTING INSTRUCTIONS

See "Spine Extension Testing"

CLINICAL PEARLS

1. The patient with strong back extensor muscles and weak hip extensor muscles can hyperextend the lumbar spine but the trunk cannot be lifted from the table.
2. The patient with weak back extensors and strong hip extensors cannot raise the trunk in extension and the lumbar lordosis is lost as the pelvis tilts posteriorly.
3. During forced full extension, flexion, lateral flexion, and rotation in different positions of the trunk, the longissimus [87] is almost always prominently active.

88. SPINALIS CAPITIS, CERVICIS, AND THORACIS

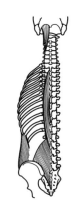

Origin
- Spinalis capitis: variable origin from the transverse processes of C7 and T1 vertebrae
- Spinalis cervicis: ligamentum nuchae, variable upper thoracic and lower cervical spinous processes
- Spinalis thoracis: variable from the spinous processes of lower thoracic and upper lumbar vertebrae

Insertion
- Spinalis capitis: between the superior and inferior nuchal lines of the occiput
- Spinalis cervicis: spinous process of the axis and variable into the spinous processes of the upper cervical vertebrae
- Spinalis thoracis: spinous processes of upper thoracic vertebrae

Roots Cervical and thoracic nerve roots

Trunk N/A

Cord N/A

Nerve Direct branches off of spinal nerve roots

Muscle Actions
- Extends the vertebral column
- Lateral flexion of the vertebral column to the same side
- Rotation to the same side

Synergists

Muscle	Nerve	Root
Iliocostalis cervicis [86]	Direct branches of spinal nerves	Cervical roots
Longissimus capitis [87]	Direct branches of spinal nerves	Cervical roots
Longissimus cervicis [87]	Direct branches of spinal nerves	Cervical roots
Semispinalis capitis [89]	Direct branches of spinal nerves	Cervical roots
Semispinalis cervicis [89]	Direct branches of spinal nerves	Cervical roots
Splenius capitis [104]	Direct branches of spinal nerves	Cervical roots
Splenius cervicis [104]	Direct branches of spinal nerves	Cervical roots
Upper trapezius (upper fibers) [1]	Spinal accessory nerve	C2-4
Iliocostalis thoracis [86]	Direct branches of spinal nerves	Cervical roots
Iliocostalis lumborum [86]	Direct branches of spinal nerves	Cervical roots
Interspinales	Direct branches of spinal nerves	Cervicothoracic roots
Longissimus thoracis [87]	Direct branches of spinal nerves	Thoracic roots

Antagonists

Muscle	Nerve	Root
Rectus capitis anticus major	Direct branch of spinal nerve	C1-2
Rectus capitis anticus minor	Direct branch of spinal nerve	C1-2
Rectus capitis lateralis	Direct branch of spinal nerve	C1-2
Longus colli	Direct branch of spinal nerve	C5-8
Scalenus anticus [108]	Direct branch of spinal nerve	C3-8
Scalenus medius [108]	Direct branch of spinal nerve	C3-8
Sternocleidomastoid [107]	Spinal accessory nerve	C2-3
Internal abdominal obliques [84]	Intercostals, iliohypogastric, ilioinguinal	T5-L1
External abdominal obliques [83]	Intercostals, iliohypogastric, ilioinguinal	T5-L1
Rectus abdominus [82]	Intercostals	T5-12

MUSCLE TESTING INSTRUCTIONS

See "Spine Extension Testing"

CLINICAL PEARLS

See "Spine Extension Testing"

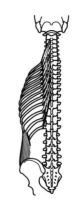

89. SEMISPINALIS CAPITIS AND CERVICIS

Origin
- Capitis
    - Transverse processes of the upper 6 or 7 thoracic and seventh cervical vertebrae
    - Articular processes of the C4-6 (variable)
- Cervicis
    - Transverse processes of the upper 6 thoracic vertebrae

Insertion
- Capitis
    - Between the superior and inferior nuchal lines of the occiput
- Cervicis
    - Cervical spinous processes (axis through C5)

Roots C4-8

Nerve Direct branches off of spinal nerves

Muscle Actions
- Semispinalis cervicis rotates the head to the opposite side
- Neck extension

Synergists

Muscle	Nerve	Root
• Iliocostalis cervicis [86]	Direct branches of spinal nerves	Cervical roots
• Longissimus capitis [87]	Direct branches of spinal nerves	Cervical roots
• Longissimus cervicis [87]	Direct branches of spinal nerves	Cervical roots
• Splenius capitis [104]	Direct branches of spinal nerves	Cervical roots
• Splenius cervicis [104]	Direct branches of spinal nerves	Cervical roots
• Upper trapezius (upper fibers) [1]	Spinal accessory nerve	C2-4
• Interspinales	Direct branches of spinal nerves	Cervicothoracic roots

Antagonists

Muscle	Nerve	Root
• Rectus capitis anticus major	Direct branch of spinal nerve	C1-2
• Rectus capitis anticus minor	Direct branch of spinal nerve	C1-2
• Rectus capitis lateralis	Direct branch of spinal nerve	C1-2
• Longus colli	Direct branch of spinal nerve	C5-8
• Scalenus anticus [108]	Direct branch of spinal nerve	C3-8
• Scalenus medius [108]	Direct branch of spinal nerve	C3-8
• Sternocleidomastoid [107]	Spinal accessory nerve	C2-3

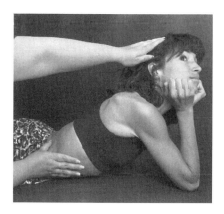

MUSCLE TESTING INSTRUCTIONS

Patient
Prone with the elbow bent and hands under the chin (sphynx position).

Tester
The tester stands at side supporting the trunk and head.

Test
"Turn your head toward me and lift your head backwards."

Pitfalls
If the neck is extended too far, the deep suboccipital muscles may be activated.

CLINICAL PEARLS

1. The upper trapezius [1] may be tested in same position by turning the head away from the tester.
2. The semispinalis capitis and cervicis [89] support the head and are noted to maintain continuous activity during upright posture.

90. MULTIFIDUS

Origin
- Transverse processes of C4-L5
- Sacrum
- Posterior superior iliac spine
- Sacroiliac ligaments

Insertion
- Spinous process of a vertebrae above the origin

Roots   Cervical, thoracic, lumbar, and sacral nerve roots

Nerve   Direct branches off of spinal nerve roots

Copyright © 1997, McGraw-Hill.

Muscle Actions
- Extends the vertebral column
- Lateral flexion of the vertebral column

Synergists

Muscle	Nerve	Root
• Iliocostalis cervicis [86]	Direct branches of spinal nerves	Cervical roots
• Iliocostalis thoracis [86]	Direct branches of spinal nerves	Thoracic roots
• Iliocostalis lumborum [86]	Direct branches of spinal nerves	Lumbar roots
• Interspinales	Direct branches of spinal nerves	C, T, L roots
• Longissimus cervicis [87]	Direct branches of spinal nerves	Cervical roots
• Longissimus thoracis [87]	Direct branches of spinal nerves	Lumbar roots
• Rotatores [91]	Direct branches of spinal nerves	C, T, L roots
• Semispinalis cervicis [89]	Direct branches of spinal nerves	Cervical roots
• Semispinalis thoracis	Direct branches of spinal nerves	Thoracic roots
• Spinalis cervicis [88]	Direct branches of spinal nerves	Cervical roots
• Spinalis thoracis [88]	Direct branches of spinal nerves	Thoracic roots
• Quadratus lumborum [85]	Direct branches of spinal nerves	T12-L1

Antagonists

Muscle	Nerve	Root
• Internal abdominal obliques [84]	Intercostals, iliohypogastric, ilioinguinal	T5-L1
• External abdominal obliques [83]	Intercostals, iliohypogastric, ilioinguinal	T5-L1
• Rectus abdominis [82]	Intercostals	T5-12

MUSCLE TESTING INSTRUCTIONS

The multifidi [90] muscles are part of the erector spinae group of muscles, thus as spine extensors they cannot be separately tested from the other muscles of this group. Hence, the same tests described above are also used for this muscle group. Like the quadratus lumborum [85], they also provide for lateral flexion of the spine, hence their action cannot be separated from that of the quadratus and thus are tested in the same fashion. See "Spine Extension Testing."

CLINICAL PEARLS

1. During needle electromyography of the paraspinals, the multifidi [90] are the desired muscles to localize, as they are theoretically innervated by the posterior primary ramus branch from the same spinal level.

91. ROTATORES

Origin
- Transverse processes of vertebrae from axis to sacrum

Insertion
- Lamina of vertebra above

Roots Cervical, thoracic, lumbar, and sacral nerve roots

Nerve Direct branches off of spinal nerve roots

Muscle Actions
- Extends the vertebral column
- Rotation to opposite side

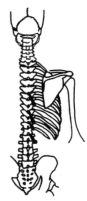

Synergists

Muscle	Nerve	Root
Iliocostalis cervicis [86]	Direct branches of spinal nerves	Cervical roots
Iliocostalis thoracis [86]	Direct branches of spinal nerves	Thoracic roots
Iliocostalis lumborum [86]	Direct branches of spinal nerves	Lumbar roots
Interspinales	Direct branches of spinal nerves	C, T, L roots
Longissimus cervicis [87]	Direct branches of spinal nerves	Cervical roots
Longissimus thoracis [87]	Direct branches of spinal nerves	Lumbar roots
Multifidus [90]	Direct branches of spinal nerves	C, T, L roots
Semispinalis cervicis [89]	Direct branches of spinal nerves	Cervical roots
Semispinalis thoracis	Direct branches of spinal nerves	Thoracic roots
Spinalis cervicis [88]	Direct branches of spinal nerves	Cervical roots
Spinalis thoracis [88]	Direct branches of spinal nerves	Thoracic roots
Quadratus lumborum [85]	Direct branches of spinal nerves	T12-L1

Antagonists

Muscle	Nerve	Root
Internal abdominal obliques [84]	Intercostals, iliohypogastric, ilioinguinal	T5-L1
External abdominal obliques [83]	Intercostals, iliohypogastric, ilioinguinal	T5-L1
Rectus abdominis [82]	Intercostals	T5-12

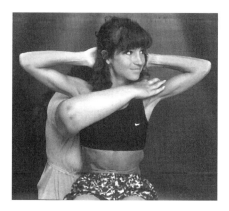

MUSCLE TESTING INSTRUCTIONS

Patient
Seated with the hands clasped behind the head.

Tester
The tester stands behind the patient and wraps the contralateral arm around the patient's neck and precordium, placing it on the patient's shoulder. The tester's thumb should be on the patient's clavicle and the fingertips on the acromion.

Test
Patient is instructed to turn the trunk toward the same side the hand is resting on shoulder with tester providing resistance.

Pitfalls
The tester's fingertips on the acromion must provide adequate resistance to backward or posterior movements for this test to be properly done.

CLINICAL PEARLS

1. This muscle will show almost continuous activity in the relaxed extended position.
2. During left-sided rotation both the left- and right-sided rotatores will be activated in the thoracic region while only the right-sided rotatores in the lumbar region will be activated.
3. The rotatores [91] lie deep to the multifidus [90] in the groove between the spinous and transverse processes and generally cannot be differentiated from the deeper fibers of the multifidus [90].

SPINE EXTENSION TESTING

CERVICAL SPINE EXTENSION

Patient

The patient is lying prone with the arms straight behind and the head hanging over the edge of the table. The patient extends the neck against the resistance of the tester's hand.

Tester

The tester uses one hand to stabilize the patient's upper thoracic area and the other hand to exert resistance against the patient's occiput as the patient attempts to extend at the neck.

Test

"Lie flat on your stomach with your arms lying behind you. Pick up your head against my hand."

Pitfalls

- If the patient's thorax is not properly stabilized, he/she might substitute thoracic spine extensors for neck extensors, thus lifting the trunk up off the table and giving the appearance of cervical spine extension.
- If the patient turns his/her head, other muscles come into play. For example, the upper trapezius [1], splenius capitis[104], splenius cervicis [104], semispinalis capitis [89], and semispinalis cervicis [89] all act as posterolateral neck extensors.
- Since factors such as tension of the anterior longitudinal ligament of the cervical spine, tightness of the ventral neck muscles, and approximation of the spinous processes can limit neck extension, the extent of the possible range of motion should be checked if there appears to be limited extension. In this way, grading the neck extensors as falsely weak can be prevented.

CLINICAL PEARLS

1. If the patient is uncomfortable in this position, use a pillow under the upper chest.
2. If still uncomfortable, attempt the test with the head lying flat on the table rather than hanging over the edge of the table.
3. Exact performance of the test may not be possible in the patient with torticollis.
4. NOTE: The iliocostalis [86] muscles are part of a group of muscles known collectively as the erector spinae muscles. These muscles act primarily as their name implies to extend the spine. Other muscles of this group include longissimus (capitis, cervicis, and thoracis) [87], the spinalis (capitis, cervicis, and thoracis) [88], the semispinalis (capitis and cervicis) [89], the multifidi [90], and the rotatori [91].

THORACIC SPINE EXTENSION

Patient

Prone with the hands clasped behind the buttocks, or the hands clasped behind the head.

Tester

If the patient has the hands clasped behind the buttocks, then the tester must use one hand to apply firm pressure to the mid-back and the other hand to apply pressure to the back of the legs. If the patient has the hands clasped behind the head, then the tester simply presses down firmly on the legs thereby stabilizing the pelvis. This indirectly fixes the hip extensors.

The muscle strength is graded as follows:

- *Normal:* Patient can raise the trunk in extension to the extent that range of motion of the back permits and can hold this position momentarily.
- *Slight weakness:* The subject can raise the trunk in extension but cannot hold the end range position even momentarily.
- *Moderate weakness:* The subject cannot raise the trunk in extension to end range position.
- *Marked weakness:* The subject cannot raise the trunk in extension at all.

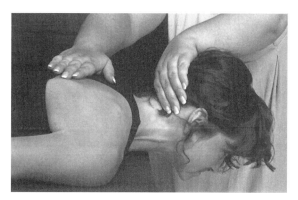

Cervical Spine Extension

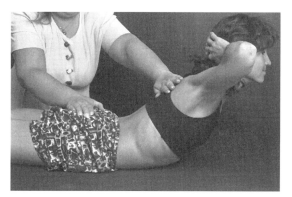

Thoracic Spine Extension

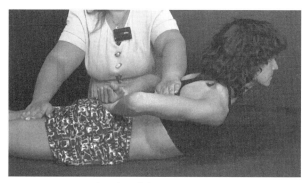

Lumbar Spine Extension

Test

"Lie flat on your stomach, clasp your hands behind your head or back, and raise your trunk up as high as possible."

Pitfalls

• In the presence of tight hip flexors, the patient will assume a position of slight lordosis of the lumbosacral spine when lying prone. Hence, the patient will be limited in the height that he/she can raise the trunk. This might then be misinterpreted as spine extensor weakness.

• In the presence of weak hip extensors, the pelvis cannot be properly stabilized. This is often erroneously interpreted as back extensor weakness. Thus, the patient will be able to hyperextend the spine (first phase) but will not be able to lift the trunk from the table (second phase).

CLINICAL PEARLS

1. Prior to performing the test, check for hip flexor tightness. If hip flexor tightness is present, then try to factor this in when determining the maximum height that the patient extends his/her trunk.

2. Prior to performing the test, check for hip extensor weakness. If the hip extensors are weak, the tester can stabilize the pelvis firmly in the direction of a posterior pelvic tilt by also using a second tester or straps to hold down the legs.

3. Marked weakness of the erector spinae muscles as a group is not seen except in connection with neuromuscular diseases. Even in some of these conditions, the erector spinae muscles are often spared.

4. NOTE: The iliocostalis [86] muscles are part of a group of muscles known collectively as the erector spinae muscles. These muscles act primarily (as their name implies) to extend the spine. Other muscles of this group include longissimus (capitis, cervicis, and thoracis) [87], the spinalis (capitis, cervicis, and thoracis) [88], the semispinalis (capitis and cervicis) [89], the multifidi [90], and the rotatori [91].

LUMBAR SPINE EXTENSION

Patient

Prone with the hands clasped behind the buttocks, or the hands clasped behind the head.

Tester

If the patient has the hands clasped behind the buttocks, then the tester must use one hand to apply firm pressure to the low-back and the other hand to apply pressure to the back of the legs. If the patient has the hands clasped behind the head, then the tester simply presses down firmly on the legs thereby stabilizing the pelvis. This indirectly fixes the hip extensors.

The muscle strength is graded as follows:

• *Normal:* Patient can raise the trunk in extension to the extent that range of motion of the back permits and can hold this position momentarily.

• *Slight weakness:* The subject can raise the trunk in extension but cannot hold the end range position even momentarily.

• *Moderate weakness:* The subject cannot raise the trunk in extension to end range position.

• *Marked weakness:* The subject cannot raise the trunk in extension at all.

Test

"Lie flat on your stomach, clasp your hands behind your head or back, and raise your trunk up as high as possible."

Pitfalls

- In the presence of tight hip flexors, the patient will assume a position of slight lordosis of the lumbosacral spine when lying prone. Hence, the patient will be limited in the height that he/she can raise the trunk. This might then be misinterpreted as spine extensor weakness.
- In the presence of weak hip extensors, the pelvis cannot be properly stabilized. This is often erroneously interpreted as back extensor weakness. Thus the patient will be able to hyperextend the spine (first phase) but will not be able to lift the trunk from the table (second phase).

CLINICAL PEARLS

1. Prior to performing the test, check for hip flexor tightness. If hip flexor tightness is present, then try to factor this in when determining the maximum height that the patient extends his/her trunk.
2. Prior to performing the test, check for hip extensor weakness. If the hip extensors are weak, the tester can stabilize the pelvis firmly in the direction of a posterior pelvic tilt by also using a second tester or straps to hold down the legs.
3. Marked weakness of the erector spinae muscles as a group is not seen except in connection with neuromuscular diseases. Even in some of these conditions, the erector spinae muscles are often spared.
4. NOTE: The iliocostalis [86] muscles are part of a group of muscles known collectively as the erector spinae muscles. These muscles act primarily (as their name implies) to extend the spine. Other muscles of this group include longissimus (capitis, cervicis, and thoracis) [87], the spinalis (capitis, cervicis, and thoracis) [88], the semispinalis (capitis and cervicis) [89], the multifidi [90], and the rotatori [91].

QUESTIONS

1. Which muscle group should be assessed for flexibility prior to testing the strength of rectus abdominis [82]?
2. Name three muscles that act synergistically with the rectus abdominis [82].
3. Name three nerves that innervate both the internal [84] and external abdominal obliques [83].
4. What are the four major functions of the internal [84] and external abdominal obliques [83]?
5. In turning the trunk to the left, name the major muscles that are acting ipsilaterally and contralaterally.

6. Describe how you would test the strength of the quadratus lumborum [85].
7. Describe two pitfalls in assessing the strength of the thoracic spine extensors?
8. Besides extending the neck, the semispinalis cervicis [89] performs what other function?
9. Describe how you would test the strength of the cervical spine extensors.
10. In the lumbar spine, the rotatores [91] have the distinction of performing what function as compared to the other spinal extensors?

CHAPTER **8**

HEAD, NECK, AND FACE

Deanna M. Janora and Marianne Sturr

92. Frontalis
93. Nasalis
94. Procerus
95. Orbicularis oculi
96. Levator palpebrae superioris
97. Orbicularis oris
98. Zygomaticus major and minor
99. Buccinator
100. Platysma/depressor anguli oris
101. Masseter
102. Temporalis
103. Medial and lateral pterygoid
104. Splenius capitis and cervicis
105. Rectus capitis posterior major and minor
106. Obliquus capitis superior and inferior
107. Sternocleidomastoid
108. Scalenes (anterior, middle, and posterior)

MUSCLES OMITTED
Anterior vertebral muscles (longus cervicis, capitis, rectus capitis anterior, lateral)
Corrugator supercilii
Depressor septi
Levator anguli oris
Risorius
Levator labii superioris
Mentalis

MUSCLE FUNCTION AT SPECIFIC JOINTS

MASTICATION
Medial pterygoid
Lateral pterygoid
Temporalis
Masseter

JAW CLOSING
  Medial pterygoid
  Temporalis
  Masseter

JAW OPENING
  Lateral pterygoid

SMILING
  Zygomaticus major
  Zygomaticus minor
  Buccinator
  Risorius

FROWNING
  Platysma
  Depressor anguli oris

92. FRONTALIS

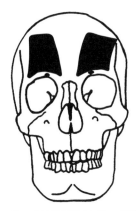

Copyright © 1997, McGraw-Hill.

Origin
- Occipital belly: short tendinous fibers from lateral two-thirds of superior nuchal line and mastoid part of temporal bone
- Frontal belly: medial fibers continuous with procerus [94] muscle, intermediate fibers blend with corrugator supercilii and orbicularis oculi [95]

Insertion
- Occipital belly: galea aponeurotica (deepest layer of scalp, tendinous layer that covers loose subaponeurotic tissue and calverium)
- Frontal belly: galea aponeurotica below coronal suture

Roots N/A

Trunk N/A

Cord N/A

Nerve
- Occipital belly: posterior auricular branch of facial nerve (CN VII)
- Frontal belly: temporal branch of facial nerve (CN VII)

Open Chain Actions
SOLO ACTION (frontalis [92])
- Raises eyebrows on either or both sides
- Wrinkles forehead horizontally

COMBINED ACTION (bilateral occipitofrontalis [92])
- Draws scalp back (as in an expression of surprise)

Synergists N/A

Antagonists

Muscle	Nerve	Branch
• Procerus [94]	Facial (CN VII)	Buccal
• Corrugator supercilii	Facial (CN VII)	Temporal

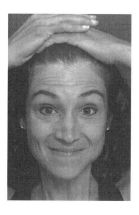

MUSCLE TESTING INSTRUCTIONS

Patient

Looks straight ahead with the face at rest.

Tester

Looks at the patient's face.

Test

"Raise your eyebrows."

Pitfalls

N/A

CLINICAL PEARLS

1. These muscles are often involved in tension headaches and referral patterns of myofascial pain.

93. NASALIS

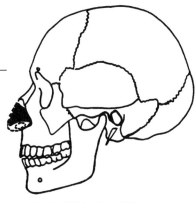

Origin
- Maxilla, above and lateral to incisor fossa

Insertion
- First insertion: skin at the lower margin in ala of the nose
- Second insertion: the tendon across the bridge of the nose, combined with the nasalis [93] from the other side

Roots N/A

Trunk N/A

Cord N/A

Nerve Buccal branch of the facial nerve (CN VII)

Open Chain Actions

SOLO ACTION N/A

COMBINED ACTION
- Widens apertures of the nostrils (flare the nostrils)

Synergists N/A

Antagonists N/A

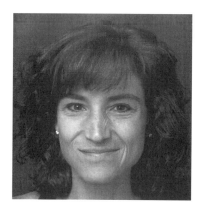

MUSCLE TESTING INSTRUCTIONS

Patient
Looks forward, the face relaxed.

Tester
Looks at the patient's face.

Test
"Flare your nostrils."

Pitfalls
The patient may be unable to voluntarily isolate its activation.

CLINICAL PEARLS

1. Asking the patient to take a slow deep breath through the nose may help accentuate this action if the patient is unable to activate this muscle voluntarily.

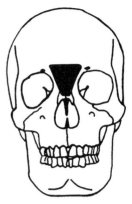

94. PROCERUS

Origin
- Lower part of nasal bone
- Upper lateral nasal cartilage

Insertion
- Skin over lower part of forehead between eyebrows

Roots N/A

Trunk N/A

Cord N/A

Nerve Buccal branch of facial nerve (CN VII)

Open Chain Actions

SOLO ACTION
- Draws down the medial angle of the eyebrows

COMBINED ACTION
- Produces vertical wrinkles over the bridge of the nose

Synergists

Muscle	Nerve	Branch
• Corrugator supercilii	Facial nerve (CN VII)	Temporal

Antagonists

Muscle	Nerve	Branch
• Frontalis [92]	Facial (CN VII)	Temporal

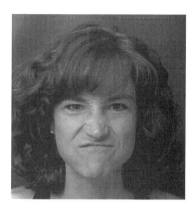

MUSCLE TESTING INSTRUCTIONS

Patient

Looks forward, the face relaxed.

Tester

Looks at the patient's face.

Test

"Wrinkle your nose."

Pitfalls

The muscle may be absent or the patient may be unable to voluntarily isolate its activation.

CLINICAL PEARLS

1. The action of this muscle gives the face an appearance of anger.

95. ORBICULARIS OCULI

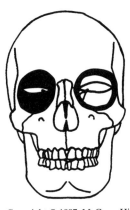

Origin
- Medial side of the orbit (nasal part of frontal bone from the frontal process of maxilla in front of lacrimal groove and from the anterior surface and borders of the medial palpebral ligament)

Insertion
- Palpebral portion: skin of upper and lower eyelids
- Orbital portion: widespread insertion in to skin of orbit, forehead, and cheek

Roots N/A

Trunk N/A

Cord N/A

Nerve Temporal and zygomatic branches of the facial nerve (CN VII)

Open Chain Actions
SOLO ACTION
- Palpebral portion: closes eyelid gently (blinking)
- Orbital portion: closes eyelid strongly (winking)
- Entire muscle: draws skin of forehead, temple, and cheek toward medial angle of the orbit

COMBINED ACTION
- Closes both eyes

Synergists N/A

Antagonists

Muscle	Nerve	Branch
• Levator palpebrae superioris [96]	Sympathetic, oculomotor (CN III)	Superior
• Frontalis [92]	Facial (CN VII)	Temporal

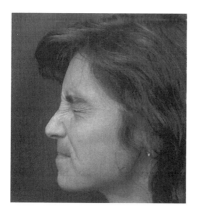

MUSCLE TESTING INSTRUCTIONS

Patient
Looks forward, the face relaxed.

Tester
Looks at the patient's face and the tester attempts to open the patient's eyelids against resistance.

Test
"Close your eyes, one at a time or together."

Pitfalls
N/A

CLINICAL PEARLS

1. If the eyes are closed tightly, it is primarily the orbital portion; whereas if the eyes are closed gently, it is primarily the palpebral portion of the orbicularis oculi [95] that is active.
2. The folds formed from the lateral angle of the eyes by the actions of this muscle may become permanent in old age and appear as "crow's feet."
3. If there is a central facial nerve injury, this muscle may not be noticeably affected due to bilateral central innervation.
4. If there is a peripheral facial nerve injury, as in Bell's palsy, this muscle will be affected on the side of the lesion, causing asymmetry of ability to close the eyelids.

96. LEVATOR PALPEBRAE SUPERIORIS

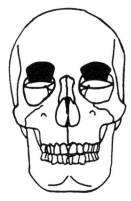

Origin
- Inferior surface of the lesser wing of the sphenoid
- Above and in front of optic canal (inside medial–superior aspect of orbit)

Insertion
- Anteriorly in the superior tarsal plate (cartilage) and skin of upper lid

Roots N/A

Trunk N/A

Cord N/A

Nerve
- Oculomotor (CN III)
- Sympathetic innervation to the smooth muscle portion from the superior cervical ganglion

Open Chain Actions
SOLO ACTION
- Opens ipsilateral eyelid

COMBINED ACTION
- Opens both eyelids

Synergists N/A

Antagonists

Muscle	Nerve	Branches
• Orbicularis oculi [95]	Facial (CN VII)	Temporal and zygomatic

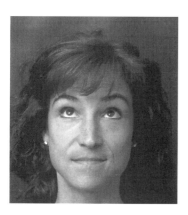

MUSCLE TESTING INSTRUCTIONS

Patient
Looks ahead with the face relaxed and the eyelids closed.

Tester
Looks at the patient's face.

Test
"Open your eyes. Raise the upper eyelid."

Pitfalls
The patient may activate the frontalis [92] muscle in addition.

CLINICAL PEARLS

1. If this muscle is paralyzed, the eyelid is held in a half-closed position.
2. This muscle is composed of voluntary skeletal muscle (superficial and deep lamellae) innervated by CN III and involuntary smooth muscle (middle lamella) innervated by the postganglionic sympathetic fibers of the superior cervical ganglion. Blocks of the sympathetic cervical ganglion, such as those done for treatment of reflex sympathetic dystrophy, will also produce a drooping eyelid on the ipsilateral side.
3. The levator palpebrae superioris [96] is continually active during waking hours *except* when closing the eyes.

97. ORBICULARIS ORIS

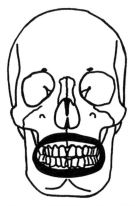

Origin
- Midline of the maxilla
- Midline of the mandible
- Deep surface of skin around the mouth

Insertion
- Skin and mucous membranes of the lips, predominantly medially

Roots N/A

Trunk N/A

Cord N/A

Nerve Buccal and mandibular branches of the facial nerve (CN VII)

Open Chain Actions
SOLO ACTION
- Deviates the lips laterally away from the side of the muscle action

COMBINED ACTION
- Closes or puckers the lips

Synergists N/A

Antagonists

Muscle	Nerve	Branch
• Buccinator [99]	Facial (CN VII)	Buccal
• Zygomaticus major [98]	Facial (CN VII)	Buccal

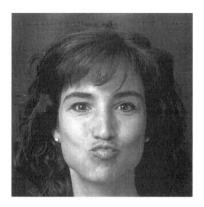

MUSCLE TESTING INSTRUCTIONS

Patient
Looks forward with the face relaxed.

Tester
Looks at the patient's face.

Test
"Pucker your lips."

Pitfalls
Be sure the patient's lips are protruding forward and not simply pursed together since this action is performed by other facial muscles.

CLINICAL PEARLS

1. With facial nerve injury (central or peripheral), weakness of the ipsilateral side of the mouth may be evident, causing drooping of the lips at rest or medial deviation of the lips with attempts to activate mouth muscles. This is due to the unopposed action of the contralateral muscles.

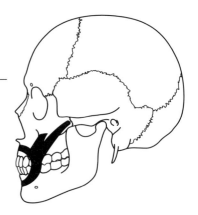

98. ZYGOMATICUS MAJOR AND MINOR

Origin
- Major: central portion of the zygomatic arch in front of the zygomatico-temporal suture and fascia of the upper part of parotid gland
- Minor: medial aspect of the zygomatic bone, behind the zygomatico-maxillary suture, often continuous with muscles of the eye such as the orbicularis oculi [95]

Insertion
- Major: skin at angle of mouth (becomes in part continuous with the orbicularis oris [97])
- Minor: lateral skin of the upper lip

Roots N/A

Trunk N/A

Cord N/A

Nerve Zygomatic and/or buccal branches of the facial nerve (CN VII)

Open Chain Actions
SOLO ACTION
- Pulls corner of mouth laterally and superiorly on same side

COMBINED ACTION
- Pulls both corners of mouth laterally and superiorly (smile)

Synergists

Muscle	Nerve	Branch
• Risorius	Facial (CN VII)	Buccal
• Buccinator [99]	Facial (CN VII)	Buccal

Antagonists

Muscle	Nerve	Branch
• Platysma [100]	Facial (CN VII)	Cervical
• Depressor anguli oris [100]	Facial (CN VII)	Mandibular

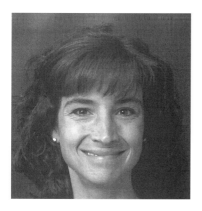

MUSCLE TESTING INSTRUCTIONS

Patient
The patient looks forward with the face relaxed.

Tester
Looks at the patient's face.

Test
"Smile."

Pitfalls
N/A

CLINICAL PEARLS

1. The zygomaticus minor [98] forms the nasolabial furrow that is deepened in expressions of sadness.
2. With facial nerve injury (central or peripheral), weakness of the ipsilateral side of the mouth may be evident, causing drooping of the lips at rest or medial deviation of the lips with attempts to activate mouth muscles. This is due to the unopposed action of the contralateral muscles.

99. BUCCINATOR

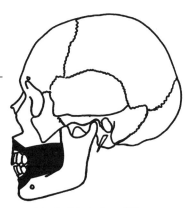

Origin
- Maxilla alongside the bony base (alveolar processes) of the posterior molar teeth
- Mandible alongside the bony base (alveolar processes) of the posterior molar teeth
- Pterygomandibular ligament

Insertion
- Angle of the mouth, blending with the orbicularis oris [97]

Roots N/A

Trunk N/A

Cord N/A

Nerve Buccal branch of facial nerve (CN VII)

Copyright © 1997, McGraw-Hill.

Open Chain Actions

SOLO ACTION
- Compresses the ipsilateral cheek and lips against teeth

COMBINED ACTION
- Purses the lips together by pulling the angles of the lips laterally

Synergists

Muscle	Nerve	Branch
• Zygomaticus major/minor [98]	Facial (CN VII)	Buccal
• Risorius	Facial (CN VII)	Buccal

Antagonists

Muscle	Nerve	Branch
• Orbicularis oris [97]	Facial (CN VII)	Buccal

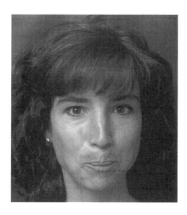

MUSCLE TESTING INSTRUCTIONS

Patient
The patient looks forward with the face relaxed.

Tester
Looks at the patient's face.

Test
"Puff up your cheeks with air then force it out by pressing cheeks against the side of your teeth."

Pitfalls
N/A

CLINICAL PEARLS

1. The buccinator [99] forms the lateral wall of the oral cavity.
2. The buccinator [99] is an accessory muscle of mastication, which holds food under the immediate pressure of the teeth.
3. With facial nerve injury (central or peripheral), weakness of the ipsilateral side of the mouth may be evident, causing drooping of the lips at rest or medial deviation of the lips with attempts to activate mouth muscles. This is due to the unopposed action of the contralateral muscles.
4. The buccal nerve, a branch of the mandibular portion of the trigeminal nerve (CN V), provides sensation to the inside of the cheek. This is not related to the buccinator [99] muscle.

100. PLATYSMA/DEPRESSOR ANGULI ORIS

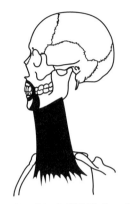

Origin
- Platysma
  - Fascia covering superior parts of the pectoralis major [9, 10]
  - Fascia covering superior parts of the deltoid [12, 13, 14]
  - Anterior thoracic wall
- Depressor anguli oris
  - Oblique line of the mandible

Insertion
- Platysma
  - Skin on the inferior and posterior aspect of the chin
  - Angle and lower part of the mouth
  - Lower border of the mandible below the oblique line
- Depressor anguli oris
  - Lateral angle of the mouth

Roots N/A

Trunk N/A

Cord N/A

Nerve
- Platysma
  - Cervical branches of the facial nerve (CN VII)
  - Mandibular branch of the facial nerve (CN VII)
- Depressor anguli oris
  - Mandibular branch of the facial nerve (CN VII)

Open Chain Actions
SOLO ACTION
- Platysma/depressor anguli oris: draws the corner of the mouth inferiorly

COMBINED ACTION
- Bilateral platysma: draws the skin over the clavicle upward toward the mandible thus increasing the diameter of the neck
- Bilateral depressor anguli oris: causes a frown

Synergists N/A

Antagonists

Muscle	Nerve	Branch
• Zygomaticus major/minor [98]	Facial (CN VII)	Buccal
• Risorius	Facial (CN VII)	Buccal

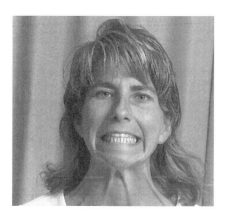

MUSCLE TESTING INSTRUCTIONS

Platysma and depressor anguli oris together:

Patient
Looks forward with the face and neck relaxed.

Tester
The tester looks at the patient's face and neck.

Test
"Pull the lower lip and angle of your mouth down and out to the side making the skin over the front of your neck tight."

Pitfalls
N/A

CLINICAL PEARLS

1. Electrodiagnostic studies have shown the platysma [100] muscle is *not* used in motions of the head and jaw or in laughing.
2. The platysma [100] can produce an expression of fear/horror.
3. The depressor anguli oris [100] can produce an expression of sadness.

101. MASSETER

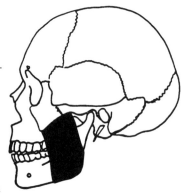

Origin
- Lower border and medial surface of the zygomatic arch (both superficial and deep portions)

Insertion
- Superficial portion: angle of the mandible and inferior half of the ramus of the mandible
- Deep portion: coronoid process of the mandible (medial to the zygomatic arch) and superior half of the ramus of the mandible

Roots N/A

Trunk N/A

Cord N/A

Nerve Masseteric, a branch from the mandibular division of trigeminal nerve (CN V)

Open Chain Actions
SOLO ACTION
- Chewing on one side of the mouth

COMBINED ACTION
- Closes the jaw

Synergists

Muscle	Nerve	Division
• Medial pterygoid [103]	Trigeminal (CN V)	Mandibular
• Temporalis [102]	Trigeminal (CN V)	Mandibular

Antagonists

Muscle	Nerve	Division
• Lateral pterygoid	Trigeminal (CN V)	Mandibular
• Gravity		
• Mylohyoid [117]	CN V	
• Geniohyoid [117]	CN X11	
• Digastric [117]	CN V	

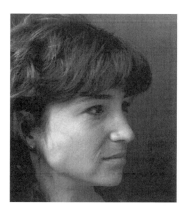

MUSCLE TESTING INSTRUCTIONS

Patient

Looks forward with the face relaxed.

Tester

The tester looks at the patient's mouth and palpates the face over the angle of the mandible.

Test

"Keep your lips open, close your jaw, and clench your teeth together."

Pitfalls

The patient can substitute the medial pterygoid [103] and temporalis [102] for this action even if the masseter [101] is paralyzed.

CLINICAL PEARLS

1. The masseter [101] is active in bruxism.
2. The masseter [101] may become dystonic after central nervous system injury causing difficulty in opening the mouth and also severe bruxism.
3. This muscle assists in biting with the incisor teeth and biting or chewing with the molar teeth.

102. TEMPORALIS

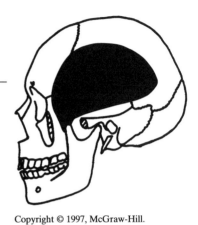

Origin
- Temporal fossa
- Surrounding fascia

Insertion
- Coronoid process of the mandible (medial to the zygomatic arch)
- Anterior border of the ramus of the mandible

Roots N/A

Trunk N/A

Cord N/A

Nerve
- Anterior and posterior deep temporal branches from the mandibular division of the trigeminal nerve (CN V)

Open Chain Actions

SOLO ACTION
- Retracts the mandible to the ipsilateral side

COMBINED ACTION
- Closes the jaw
- Retracts the mandible

Synergists

Muscle	Nerve	Division
• Medial pterygoid [103]	Trigeminal (CN V)	Mandibular
• Masseter [101]	Trigeminal (CN V)	Mandibular

Antagonists

Muscle	Nerve	Division
• Lateral pterygoid [103]	Trigeminal (CN V)	Mandibular
• Gravity		

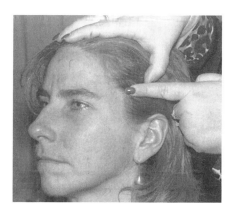

MUSCLE TESTING INSTRUCTIONS

Patient
Looks forward with the face relaxed.

Tester
The tester looks at the patient's jaw and mouth while palpating the face over the temples.

Test
"Keep your lips open, close your jaw, and clench your teeth together."

Pitfalls
It is often difficult to isolate this muscle from its two main synergists, the medial pterygoid [103] and masseter [101].

CLINICAL PEARLS

1. The temporalis [102] is often involved in "temporomandibular joint syndrome" (TMJ), tension type headache, and referral of myofascial pain.
2. This muscle assists in biting or chewing with the molar teeth.
3. The temporalis [102] may become dystonic after central nervous system injury causing difficulty in opening the mouth.

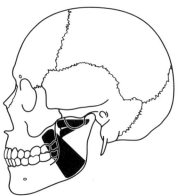

103. MEDIAL AND LATERAL PTERYGOID

Origin
- Medial: medial surface of the lateral pterygoid plate
- Lateral
  - Superior head: lateral surface of the great wing of the sphenoid
  - Inferior head: lateral surface of the lateral pterygoid plate

Insertion
- Medial: inferior and posterior aspects of the medial surface of the ramus and angle of the mandible
- Lateral (both heads): anterior part of the condyle of the mandible and anterior margin of the articular disc of the temporomandibular joint

Roots N/A

Trunk N/A

Cord N/A

Nerve
- Medial: medial pterygoid, a branch of the mandibular division of the trigeminal nerve (CN V)
- Lateral: lateral pterygoid, a branch of the mandibular division of the trigeminal nerve (CN V)

Open Chain Actions

SOLO ACTION
- Medial: chewing on one side of the mouth
- Lateral: moves the mandible from side to side

COMBINED ACTION
- Medial: closes the mouth
- Lateral: opens the mouth and protrudes the mandible forward

Synergists

Muscle	Nerve	Division
Medial pterygoid [103]		
• Temporalis [102]	Trigeminal (CN V)	Mandibular
• Masseter [101]	Trigeminal (CN V)	Mandibular
Lateral pterygoid [103]: to protrude jaw, prevents jaw-opening motion (rotation of TMJ)		
• Medial pterygoid [103]	Trigeminal (CN V)	Mandibular
• Temporalis [102]	Trigeminal (CN V)	Mandibular
• Masseter [101]	Trigeminal (CN V)	Mandibular
Lateral pterygoid [103]: to open the jaw		
• Gravity		

Antagonists

Muscle	Nerve	Division
Medial pterygoid [103]		
• Lateral pterygoid [103]	Trigeminal (CN V)	Mandibular
• Gravity		
Lateral pterygoid [103]: jaw opening		
• Medial pterygoid [103]	Trigeminal (CN V)	Mandibular
• Masseter [101]	Trigeminal (CN V)	Mandibular
• Temporalis [102]	Trigeminal (CN V)	Mandibular

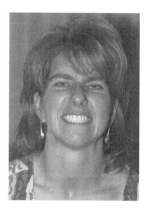

MUSCLE TESTING INSTRUCTIONS

Patient

Looks forward with the face and mouth relaxed.

Tester

The tester looks at the patient's face and mouth.

Test

"Keep your lips open (to better observe teeth) and close your mouth/clench your teeth together."

Pitfalls

N/A

CLINICAL PEARLS

1. Only one muscle opens the mouth, whereas three help to close it.
2. The medial pterygoid [103] assists in biting with the incisor teeth and biting or chewing with the molar teeth.
3. The medial pterygoid [103] may become dystonic after central nervous system injury causing difficulty in opening the mouth.

104. SPLENIUS CAPITIS AND CERVICIS

Origin:
- Capitis
  - Lower half of the ligamentum nuchae
  - Spinous processes of C7 and T1, 2, 3, and possibly T4.
- Cervicis
  - Spinous processes of T3-6

Insertion:
- Capitis
  - Lateral mastoid process
  - Occipital bone laterally
- Cervicis
  - Transverse processes of C1, 2, and maybe C3, 4

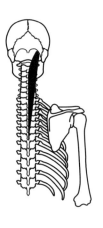

Roots N/A

Trunk N/A

Cord N/A

Nerve:
- Capitis: dorsal rami of the middle cervical spinal nerves (C3-4, variable)
- Cervicis: dorsal rami of the inferior cervical spinal nerves (C4-8, variable)

Open Chain Actions

SOLO ACTION: Capitis and cervicis act together
- Rotation of the head and neck ipsilaterally
- Lateral flexion of the neck ipsilaterally

COMBINED ACTION:
- Extension of neck

Synergists

Muscle	Nerve	Root
Lateral flexion		
• Anterior vertebral muscles	Ventral rami	C1-4
• Ipsilateral sternocleidomastoid [107]	Spinal accessory (CN XI)	C2-3
• Ipsilateral scalenes [108]	Ventral rami	C3-8
• Ipsilateral obliquus capitis superior [106]	Suboccipital	C1-2
Rotation		
• Contralateral sternocleidomastoid [107]	Spinal accessory (CN XI)	C2-3
• Ipsilateral rectus capitis posterior major [105]	Suboccipital	C1-2
• Ipsilateral obliquus capitis inferior [106]	Suboccipital	C1-2
• Ipsilateral transverse spinal muscles	Dorsal rami	Local
• Ipsilateral scalene (primarily anterior) [108]	Ventral rami	C3-8
Extension		
• Suboccipital muscles (all)	Suboccipital	C1-2
• Transverse spinal muscles (all)	Dorsal rami	Local

Antagonists

Muscle	Nerve	Root
Lateral Flexion		
• Contralateral sternocleidomastoid [107]	Spinal accessory (CN XI)	C2-3
• Contralateral scalenes [108]	Ventral rami	C3-8
• Contralateral obliquus capitis superior [106]	Suboccipital	C1-2
Rotation		
• Ipsilateral sternocleidomastoid [107]	Spinal accessory (CN XI)	C2-3
• Contralateral rectus capitis posterior major [105]	Suboccipital	C1-2
• Contralateral transverse spinal muscles	Dorsal rami	Local
• Contralateral scalene [108]	Ventral rami	C3-8
Extension		
• Anterior vertebral muscles	Ventral rami	C1-4
• Sternocleidomastoid [107]	Spinal accessory (CN XI)	C2-3
• Scalenes [108]	Ventral rami	C3-8

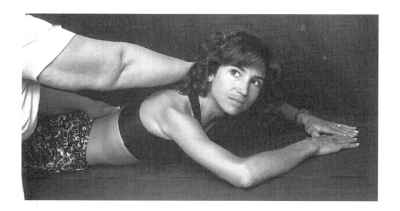

MUSCLE TESTING INSTRUCTIONS

Patient
Looks forward with the head and neck relaxed.

Tester
The tester looks at the patient's head and neck.

Test
Right muscles: "Turn your head to the right side."
Left muscles: "Turn your head to the left side."
Bilateral muscles: "Tilt your head back and look up at the ceiling."

Pitfalls
It is usually not possible to isolate the splenius [104] from other neck muscles with the same action.

CLINICAL PEARLS

1. Cervical lordosis will be increased if the splenius [104] muscles contract bilaterally and symmetrically.
2. Deep to the trapezius [1,2,3] and rhomboids [4] (superficial back muscles), the muscle fibers of the splenius [104] group run in a medial to lateral direction as they pass superiorly (the opposite direction of superficial back muscles).
3. These muscles are frequently involved in cervical dystonia and are commonly treated with chemodenervation.

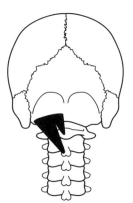

105. RECTUS CAPITIS POSTERIOR MAJOR AND MINOR

Origin
- Major: spinous process of the axis
- Minor: posterior tubercle of the atlas

Insertion
- Major: middle inferior nuchal line and the occipital bone
- Minor: medial part of the inferior nuchal line and the occiptal bone

Roots N/A

Trunk N/A

Cord N/A

Nerve Dorsal rami of C1 (Suboccipital nerve) and C2

Open Chain Actions
SOLO ACTION
- Rotates the head and neck ipsilaterally (major only)

COMBINED ACTION
- Extends the head at the occipitoatlanto joint (C0-1), as in nodding the head

Synergists

Muscle	Nerve	Root
• Contralateral sternocleidomastoid [107]	Spinal accessory (CN XI)	C2-3
• Ipsilateral splenius capitis and cervicis [104]	Dorsal rami	Local
• Ipsilateral obliquus capitis inferior [106]	Suboccipital	C1-2
• Ipsilateral transverse spinal muscles	Dorsal rami	Local
• Ipsilateral scalene (primarily anterior) [108]	Ventral rami	C3-8
• Splenius capitis and cervicis [104]	Dorsal rami	Local
• Transverse spinal muscles (all)	Dorsal rami	Local

Antagonists

Muscle	Nerve	Root
• Ipsilateral sternocleidomastoid [107]	Spinal accessory (CN XI)	C2-3
• Contralateral splenius capitis and cervicis [104]	Dorsal rami	Local
• Contralateral transverse spinal muscles	Dorsal rami	Local
• Contralateral scalene	Ventral rami	C3-8
• Anterior vertebral muscles	Ventral rami	C1-4
• Sternocleidomastoid [107]	Spinal Accessory (CN XI)	C2-3
• Scalenes [108]	Ventral rami	C3-8
• Splenius capitis and cervicis [104]	Dorsal rami	Local

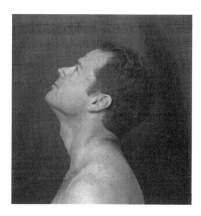

MUSCLE TESTING INSTRUCTIONS

Patient
Looks forward with the head and neck relaxed in a neutral position.

Tester
For extension movement: the tester stands on the side of the patient while looking at the head and neck.

For rotation and lateral flexion: the tester stands in front of the patient while looking at the head and neck.

Test
Rectus capitis posterior major and minor: "Tilt your head back to look at the ceiling."

Rectus capitis posterior major: "Turn your head to the right and then left" (for each side of the muscle separately).

Pitfalls
This muscle group cannot be isolated from other muscles that extend and rotate the head.

CLINICAL PEARLS

1. Simultaneous contraction of the anterior and posterior cervical spine muscle groups maintain the neck in a rigid neutral position, such as when one is balancing an object on top of one's head.

106. OBLIQUUS CAPITIS SUPERIOR
AND INFERIOR

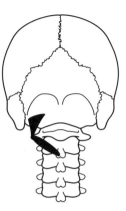

Origin
- Obliquus capitis superior: transverse process of the atlas
- Obliquus capitis inferior: spinous process of the axis

Insertion
- Obliquus capitis superior: occipital bone above the outer part of the inferior nuchal line (overlaps with the insertion on the rectus capitis posterior major [105])
- Obliquus capitis inferior: transverse process of the atlas

Roots N/A

Trunk N/A

Cord N/A

Nerve Dorsal rami of C1 (suboccipital nerve) and C2

Open Chain Actions
SOLO ACTION
- Ipsilateral rotation of the neck at the C1-2 joint (inferior only)
- Ipsilateral lateral flexion of the head at the C0-1 joint (superior only)

COMBINED ACTION
- Extends the head at the occipitoatlanto joint (C0-1) (superior only)

Synergists

Muscle	Nerve	Root
• Anterior vertebral muscles	Ventral rami	C1-4
• Ipsilateral sternocleidomastoid [107]	Spinal accessory (CN XI)	C2-3
• Ipsilateral scalenes [108]	Ventral rami	C3-8
• Contralateral sternocleidomastoid [107]	Spinal accessory (CN XI)	C2-3
• Ipsilateral splenius capitis and cervicis [104]	Dorsal rami	Local
• Ipsilateral obliquus capitis inferior [106]	Suboccipital	C1-2
• Ipsilateral transverse spinal muscles	Dorsal rami	Local
• Ipsilateral scalene (primarily anterior) [108]	Ventral rami	C3-8
• Splenius capitis and cervicis [104]	Dorsal rami	Local
• Transverse spinal muscles (all)	Dorsal rami	Local

Antagonists

Muscle	Nerve	Root
• Contralateral sternocleidomastoid [107]	Spinal accessory (CN XI)	C2-3
• Contralateral scalenes (all three) [108]	Ventral rami	C3-8
• Ipsilateral sternocleidomastoid [107]	Spinal accessory (CN XI)	C2-3
• Contralateral splenius capitis and cervicis [104]	Dorsal rami	Local
• Contralateral transverse spinal muscles	Dorsal rami	Local
• Anterior vertebral muscles	Ventral rami	C1-4
• Sternocleidomastoid [107]	Spinal accessory (CN XI)	C2-3
• Scalenes [108]	Ventral rami	C3-8
• Splenius capitis and cervicis [104]	Dorsal rami	Local

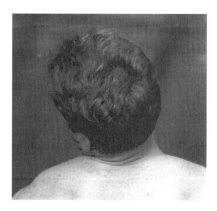

MUSCLE TESTING INSTRUCTIONS

Patient
Looks forward with the head and neck relaxed in a neutral position.

Tester
For extension movement: the tester stands on the side of the patient while looking at the head and neck.

For rotation and lateral flexion: the tester stands in front of the patient while looking at the head and neck.

Test
Obliquus capitis superior: "Tilt your head back to look at the ceiling and bring your ear toward your shoulder."

Obliquus capitis inferior: "Turn your head to the right then the left, as if to shake your head 'no'."

Pitfalls
This muscle group cannot be isolated from the other muscles that extend and rotate the head.

CLINICAL PEARLS

1. Simultaneous contraction of the anterior and posterior cervical spine muscle groups maintains the neck in a rigid neutral position, such as when one is balancing an object on top of one's head.
2. The obliquus capitis inferior [106] muscle is important in maintaining the integrity of the atlantoaxial joint (C1-2), both at rest and during movement.

107. STERNOCLEIDOMASTOID

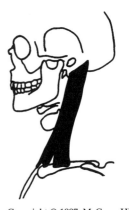

Origin
- Tendinous head: sternum (manubrium sterni)
- Muscular head: medial one-third of the clavicle

Insertion
- Mastoid process (behind the ear)

Roots N/A

Trunk N/A

Cord N/A

Nerve
- Motor: spinal accessory nerve (CN XI)
- Sensory: C2 and perhaps C3

Open Chain Actions
SOLO ACTION
- Turns the head to the opposite side (contralateral rotation)
- Ipsilateral lateral flexion/side bending

COMBINED ACTION
- Powerfully flexes the head and neck

Closed Chain Actions
If the head is fixed, the sternocleidomastoid [107] is able to raise the clavicle and sternum (acts as an accessory muscle of respiration)

Synergists

Muscle	Nerve	Root
• Ipsilateral obliquus capitis superior [106]	Suboccipital	C1-2
• Ipsilateral scalenes (all three) [108]	Ventral rami	C3-8
• Ipsilateral splenius capitis and cervicis [104]	Dorsal rami	Local
• Contralateral rectus capitis posterior major [105]	Suboccipital	C1-2
• Contralateral splenius capitis and cervicis [104]	Dorsal rami	Local
• Contralateral obliquus capitis inferior [106]	Suboccipital	C1-2
• Contralateral transverse spinal muscles	Dorsal rami	Local
• Contralateral scalene (primarily anterior) [108]	Ventral rami	C3-8
• Anterior vertebral muscles	Ventral rami	C1-4
• Scalenes [108]	Ventral rami	C3-8

Antagonists

Muscle	Nerve	Root
• Ipsilateral rectus capitis posterior major [105]	Suboccipital	C1-2
• Ipsilateral splenius capitis and cervicis [104]	Dorsal rami	Local
• Ipsilateral obliquus capitis inferior [106]	Suboccipital	C1-2
• Ipsilateral transverse spinal muscles	Dorsal rami	Local
• Ipsilateral scalene [108]	Ventral rami	C3-8
• Contralateral obliquus capitis superior [106]	Suboccipital	C1-2
• Contralateral scalenes [108]	Ventral rami	C3-8
• Contralateral splenius capitis and cervicis [104]	Dorsal rami	Local
• Splenius capitis and cervicis [104]	Dorsal rami	Local
• Transverse spinal muscles (all)	Dorsal rami	Local
• Suboccipital muscles	Suboccipital	C1-2

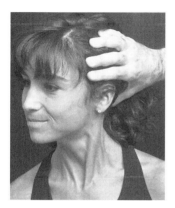

MUSCLE TESTING INSTRUCTIONS

Patient
Technique 1: While standing, the patient looks forward with the head and neck relaxed.
Technique 2: While supine, the patient lies flat on the back with the arms overhead.

Tester
Technique 1: The tester looks at the patient's head and neck with the hand over one side of the face.
Technique 2: The tester looks at the head with one hand on the patient's forehead.

Test
Technique 1: "Turn your head to the side and then push back against my hand in the opposite direction."
Technique 2: "Lift your head off of the table and don't allow me to push it down."

Pitfalls
N/A

CLINICAL PEARLS

1. If the sternocleidomastoid [107] becomes dystonic, it may cause the painful, disabling condition known as torticollis.
2. Contraction of the sternocleidomastoid [107] may increase the cervical lordosis by causing head extension relative to the cervical spine and cervical flexion relative to the thoracic spine.

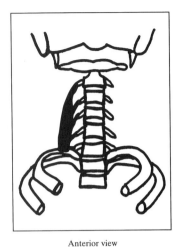
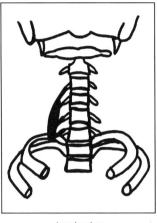
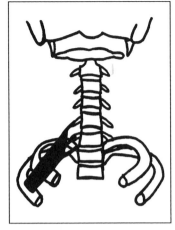

Anterior view

Anterior view

Anterior view

108. SCALENES (ANTERIOR, MIDDLE, AND POSTERIOR)

Origin
- Anterior: anterior tubercles of the transverse processes of C3-6
- Middle: anterior tubercles of the transverse process of C2-7
- Posterior: transverse processes of C4-6

Insertion
- Anterior: undersurface of first rib toward the sternal attachment
- Middle: first rib
- Posterior: lateral aspect of second rib

Roots N/A

Trunk N/A

Cord N/A

Nerve Ventral rami of the cervical nerves corresponding to the levels of origin (C3-8)

Open Chain Actions
Solo Action
- Ipsilateral side bending of the neck
- Ipsilateral rotation of the neck

Combined Action
- Fixes the first 2 ribs in quiet inspiration
- Raises the first 2 ribs in forced inspiration
- Flexes the neck forward

Synergists

Muscle	Nerve	Root
• Ipsilateral obliquus capitis superior [106]	Suboccipital	C1-2
• Ipsilateral sternocleidomastoid [107]	Spinal accessory (CN XI)	C2-3
• Ipsilateral splenius capitis and cervicis [104]	Dorsal rami	Local
• Ipsilateral rectus capitis post. major [105]	Suboccipital	C1-2
• Ipsilateral obliquus capitis inferior [106]	Suboccipital	C1-2
• Ipsilateral transverse spinal muscles	Dorsal rami	Local
• Contralateral sternocleidomastoid [107]	Spinal accessory (CN XI)	C2-3
• Anterior vertebral muscles	Ventral rami	C1-4

Antagonists

Muscle	Nerve	Root
• Contralateral obliquus capitis superior/inferior[106]	Suboccipital	C1-2
• Contralateral scalenes [108]	Ventral rami	C3-8
• Contralateral splenius capitis and cervicis [104]	Dorsal rami	Local
• Contralateral rectus capitis post. major [105]	Suboccipital	C1-2
• Contralateral transverse spinal muscles	Dorsal rami	Local
• Ipsilateral sternocleidomastoid [107]	Spinal accessory (CN XI)	C2-3
• Ipsilateral splenius capitis and cervicis [104]	Dorsal rami	Local
• Transverse spinal muscles (all)	Dorsal rami	Local

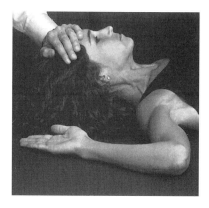

MUSCLE TESTING INSTRUCTIONS

Patient
The patient lies flat on the back with the arms overhead.

Tester
The tester stands at the patient's head with the hand over the forehead.

Test
"Lift your head off the table and don't let me push it down."

Pitfalls
The sternocleidomastoid [107] may substitute for the scalenes [108].

CLINICAL PEARLS

1. The anterior and middle scalenes [108] are separated from each other by the brachial plexus and subclavian artery.
2. The brachial plexus may be stretched over the first rib or between the anterior and middle scalenes [108] (especially if they have increased tone) and cause "scalene anticus syndrome." The symptoms of this are worsened if the shoulder is held in a lowered position such as when carrying something heavy in that hand.

QUESTIONS

1. Name the cervical spine muscle that helps to prevent neck flexion, such as in a "whiplash" type of injury.
2. Name the muscle that causes contralateral rotation of the head.
3. Name the muscle that causes ipsilateral rotation of the head.
4. If the right sternocleidomastoid [107] is hypertonic, the patient will present with their head in what position?
5. Name the four major muscles of mastication and their innervation.

6. Name the single muscle primarily responsible for opening the jaw.
7. Name the three muscles primarily responsible for closing the jaw.
8. What muscle has an insertion on the articular disc of the temporomandibular joint?
9. What muscles are responsible for the expression of smiling?
10. What muscles are responsible for the expression of frowning?

CHAPTER 9

MUSCLES OF RESPIRATION

Sally Ann Holmes

109. Diaphragm
110. External Intercostals
111. Internal Intercostals

The respiratory muscles elevate and lower the ribs, in a cyclic manner, resulting in inspiration and expiration to maintain arterial blood gases within a normal physiologic range under varying conditions from rest to extreme exertion. Due to a large cardiopulmonary reserve, homeostasis is usually maintained in spite of severe lung disease or respiratory muscle weakness. Respiratory insufficiency or failure, which results in abnormal arterial blood gas tensions, occurs after the work of breathing exceeds this reserve. Without careful assessment of respiratory muscle function, significant weakness may go undetected.

The muscles of respiration can be divided into the two following groups: muscles of inspiration which include the diaphragm [109], external intercostals [110], serratus posterior superior, and accessory muscles of inspiration; and the muscles of expiration that include the abdominal muscles [82,83,84], internal intercostals [111], transversus thoracis, and serratus posterior inferior. In general, inspiratory muscles elevate the ribs and expiratory muscles lower the ribs. Except for the accessory muscles of inspiration, manual motor testing cannot be performed on the muscles of respiration; therefore, other methods of assessment of respiratory muscle function will be discussed in this chapter. Pulmonary function tests, which are useful in assessment of respiratory muscle strength, include lung volumes, maximal static respiratory pressures, flow/volume curves, and volume/time curves. See Table 9-1 for definitions of commonly used pulmonary function tests.

Disorders affecting respiratory muscle function can generally be classified as obstructive or restrictive in pattern. In obstructive pattern disorders there is intrinsic lung involvement with a ventilation/perfusion mismatch resulting in impaired oxygenation. Examples of obstructive pattern disorders include emphysema, chronic bronchitis, asthma, cystic fibrosis, and bronchiectasis. In restrictive pattern disorders there is a mechanical or bellows dysfunction resulting in impaired ventilation. Examples of restrictive pattern disorders include neuromuscular diseases with respiratory muscle weakness such as Duchenne muscular dystrophy, postpoliomyelitis syndrome and amyotrophic lateral sclerosis; paralysis of the respiratory muscles due to traumatic tetraplegia or Guillain-Barré syndrome; and distortions of the thoracic cage due to kyphoscoliosis, or ankylosing spondylitis. Refer to Table 9-2 for characteristic alterations in pulmonary function tests for obstructive versus restrictive pattern disorders.

Table 9-1
Pulmonary Function Studies

Forced Vital Capacity (FVC): The amount of air moved when lungs are forcefully expanded after maximal expiration

Tidal Volume (TV): The amount of air moved in normal inspiratory effort

Total Lung Capacity (TLC): The amount of air contained within the lungs at the end of maximal inspiration

Functional Residual Capacity (FRC): The amount of air in the lungs at the end of normal expiration

Residual Volume (RV): The amount of air in the lungs at the end of maximal expiration

FEV_1: Forced Expiratory Volume in one second

Minute Volume: Tidal volume times rate of breathing per minute

Maximal Static Inspiratory Pressure (P$_I$max): Static pressure measured near RC after maximal expiration

Maximal Static Expiratory Pressure (P$_E$max): Static pressure measured near TLC after maximal inspiration

Maximal Voluntary Ventilation (MVV): Total volume of air expired during 12-second period of patient breathing as fast and as hard as possible; expressed in L/min

Peak Cough Flow: The amount of air flow during maximal cough expressed in L/second

Table 9-2
Characteristic Alterations in Pulmonary Function Tests

	Obstructive Pattern	*Restrictive Pattern*
FEV_1	↓	↓
FVC	↓	↓
Airflow (FEV_1/FVC, %)	↓	↔/↑
Airflow response to bronchodilators	↑/↔	↔
TLC	↑/↔	↓
FRC	↑	↓/↔
RV	↑/↔	↓/↔
MVV	↓	↓
Lung compliance	↔/↓	↓

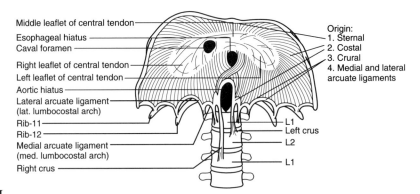

Middle leaflet of central tendon
Esophageal hiatus
Caval foramen
Right leaflet of central tendon
Left leaflet of central tendon
Aortic hiatus
Lateral arcuate ligament
(lat. lumbocostal arch)
Rib-11
Rib-12
Medial arcuate ligament
(med. lumbocostal arch)
Right crus

Origin:
1. Sternal
2. Costal
3. Crural
4. Medial and lateral
arcuate ligaments

L1
Left crus
L2
L1

109. DIAPHRAGM

Origin Thoracic outlet in three portions
- Sternal: posterior aspect of xiphoid process
- Costal: inner surfaces costal cartilages of ribs 7 to 12
- Lumbar: right and left crura that blend with the anterior longitudinal ligament of the first three lumbar vertebrae and the medial and lateral arcuate ligaments (lumbocostal arches)

Insertion: • 3-Leafed central tendon below the pericardium

Roots C3-5 (Primarily C4)

Nerve Right and left phrenic nerves

Actions: • As the diaphragm contracts, the domes descend expanding the thoracic cavity by increasing the longitudinal dimension of the chest, elevating the lower ribs and displacing the abdominal contents. This action decreases the pressure within the thoracic cavity and air enters the lungs because of higher atmospheric pressure.

Synergists Muscles of inspiration

Muscle	Nerve	Root
• External intercostals [110]	Intercostal nerves	T1-11
• Serratus posterior superior	Ventral rami	T1-4
Accessory muscles of inspiration		
• Scalenes (anterior, medial, posterior) [108]	Ventral rami	C3-8
• Sternocleidomastoid [107]	Cranial nerve XI, ventral rami	C2-3
• Pectoralis major and minor [9, 10, 11]	Medial and lateral pectoral nerve	C5-T1
• Trapezius [1, 2, 3]	Cranial nerve XI, ventral rami	C2-4

Antagonists Muscles of expiration

Muscle	Nerve	Root
• Internal intercostals [111]	Intercostal nerves	T1-T11
• Transversus thoracis	Intercostal nerves	T1-T11
• Serratus posterior inferior	Ventral rami	T9-T12
Abdominal muscles		
• Rectus abdominis [82]	Thoracoabdominal branches	T5-12
• External oblique [83]	Thoracoabdominal branches	T5-L1
• Internal oblique [84]	Thoracoabdominal branches	T5-L1
• Transverse abdominis	Thoracoabdominal branches	T7-L1

RESPIRATORY MUSCLE TESTING

The diaphragm is the primary muscle of inspiration. Vital capacity (FVC) and maximal inspiratory pressure (PI_{max}) are good indicators of inspiratory muscle strength. Vital capacity is measured with a spirometer. The patient is instructed to inspire maximally then exhale as much air as possible; slow maximal exhale measures VC, and rapid maximal exhale measures forced vital capacity (FVC). PI_{max}, also known as negative inspiratory pressure (NIP), is measured after maximal expiration at residual volume.

Pitfalls

1. Failure to measure lung volumes in both supine and seated positions in persons with neuromuscular disorders or spinal cord injury.
2. Poor effort due to cognitive status, pain, or anxiety during pulmonary function testing.

CLINICAL PEARLS

1. Respiratory muscle weakness or paralysis results in a mechanical disorder (bellows dysfunction) resulting in impaired ventilation. Measurement of lung volumes reveals a restrictive pattern. Airflow responses are variable.
2. The most sensitive indicator of respiratory muscle weakness is reduction in maximal static respiratory pressures.
3. Bedside predictors of extubation success in adult patient:
   FVC > 1 L
   $PI_{max} < -20$ cmH$_2$O
   Peak cough flow (PCF) > 3 L/second (J. Bach, 1994)
4. The portion of the diaphragm directly apposed to the inner aspect of the lower rib cage is known as the zone of apposition. As the dome of the diaphragm contracts during inspiration, it descends causing an increase in intraabdominal pressure. This increase in intraabdominal pressure in the zone of apposition is transmitted to the lower ribs and results in elevation of these ribs. The zone of apposition decreases with loss of passive recoil of the ventral abdominal wall or with increasing lung volumes that occur with spinal cord injury or COPD, respectively.
5. In persons with neuromuscular disorders or spinal cord injury, spirometry should be performed in both supine and seated positions. In persons with neuromuscular disorders who have diaphragmatic weakness, lung volumes are lower in the supine position due to increased work of breathing required to move the diaphragm against the abdominal contents and overcome gravity. Due to lack of recoil of the abdominal muscles in persons with spinal cord injury, lung volumes are lower in the seated position.
6. Symptoms of chronic alveolar hypoventilation due to respiratory muscle weakness are nonspecific and include the following: fatigue, sleep disturbances, morning headaches, anorexia, depression, and weight loss.
7. Mechanical ventilation (delivered noninvasively or via an indwelling tracheostomy) is the treatment of choice for respiratory insufficiency due to respiratory muscle weakness. Assisted ventilation provides respiratory muscle rest, thus decreasing the energy expenditure of the ventilatory muscles. A weaning protocol should include progressively increasing time off mechanical ventilatory support with complete rest between work periods.
8. The upper airway muscles that include the mouth, tongue, palate, and larynx are important for keeping the airway open during inspiration.

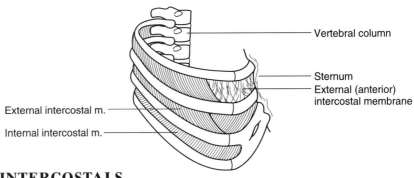

External intercostal m.

Internal intercostal m.

Vertebral column

Sternum

External (anterior) intercostal membrane

110. EXTERNAL INTERCOSTALS

Origin
- Lower border ribs 1 to 11; fibers run caudad and medially

Insertion
- Upper border of rib 2 to 12 below

Roots T1-11

Nerve Segmentally innervated by the intercostal nerves

Actions
- Elevate ribs expanding the thoracic cavity (inspiration)

Synergists Muscles of inspiration

Muscle	Nerve	Root
• Diaphragm [109]	Phrenic	C3-5
• Serratus posterior superior	Ventral rami	T1-4
Accessory muscles of inspiration		
• Scalenes (anterior, medial, posterior) [108]	Ventral rami	C3-8
• Sternocleidomastoid [107]	Cranial nerve XI, ventral rami	C2-3
• Pectoralis major and minor [9, 10, 11]	Medial and latateral pectoral nerve	C5-T1
• Trapezius [1, 2, 3]	Cranial nerve XI, ventral rami	C2-4

Antagonists Muscles of expiration

Muscle	Nerve	Root
• Internal intercostals [111]	Intercostal nerves	T1-11
• Transversus thoracis	Intercostal nerves	T1-11
• Serratus posterior inferior	Ventral rami	T9-12
Abdominal Muscles		
• Rectus abdominis [82]	Thoracoabdominal branches	T5-12
• External oblique [83]	Thoracoabdominal branches	T5-L1
• Internal oblique [84]	Thoracoabdominal branches	T5-L1
• Transverse abdominis	Thoracoabdominal branches	T7-L1

RESPIRATORY MUSCLE TESTING

Test

There are no pulmonary function tests that isolate external intercostal muscle function; however FVC and PI_{max} are good indicators of inspiratory muscle strength.

Pitfalls

Refer to sections in diaphram [109].

CLINICAL PEARLS

1. Refer to sections in diaphragm [109].

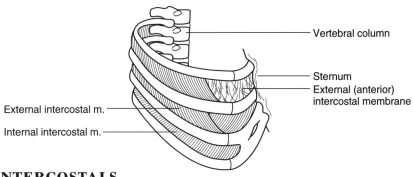

Vertebral column

Sternum
External (anterior)
intercostal membrane

External intercostal m.

Internal intercostal m.

111. INTERNAL INTERCOSTALS

Origin
- Costal cartilage and costal groove of ribs 1 to 11; fibers run caudad and laterally

Insertion
- Upper border of ribs 2 to 12 below

Roots T1-11

Nerve Segmentally innervated by intercostal nerves

Actions
- Depress ribs (expiration)

Synergists Muscles of expiration

Muscle	Nerve	Root
• Transversus thoracis	Intercostal nerves	T1-11
• Serratus posterior inferior	Ventral rami	T9-12
Abdominal muscles		
• Rectus abdominis [82]	Thoracoabdominal branches	T5-12
• External oblique [83]	Thoracoabdominal branches	T5-L1
• Internal oblique [84]	Thoracoabdominal branches	T5-L1
• Transverse abdominis	Thoracoabdominal branches	T7-L1

Antagonists Muscles of inspiration

Muscle	Nerve	Root
• Diaphragm [109]	Phrenic	C3-5
• Serratus posterior superior	Ventral rami	T1-4
Accessory muscles of inspiration		
• Scalenes (anterior, medial, posterior) [108]	Ventral rami	C3-8
• Sternocleidomastoid [107]	Cranial nerve XI, ventral rami	C2-3
• Pectoralis major and minor [9, 10, 11]	Medial and lateral pectoral nerve	C5-T1
• Trapezius [1, 2, 3]	Cranial nerve XI, ventral rami	C2-4

RESPIRATORY MUSCLE TESTING

There are no pulmonary function tests that isolate internal intercostal muscle function; however, PCF, PE_{max}, and FEV_1 are good indicators of expiratory muscle strength. A flowmeter is used to measure PCF during cough. This measure should be obtained during assisted cough if needed. PE_{max} is measured at total lung capacity (TLC). FEV_1 is a measure of forced expiratory volume in one second. Remember that the abdominal muscles are the principal muscles of forced expiration.

Pitfalls

Interpretation of pulmonary function tests of persons with respiratory muscle weakness or paralysis is based on predicted values obtained from studies of healthy persons. (Example: finding of FEV_1 40 percent predicted value in a 26-year-old patient with T5 paraplegia interpreted as obstructive pulmonary dysfunction; the patient most likely has a "functional obstruction" due to paralyzed abdominal muscles rather than obstructive pulmonary disease.)

CLINICAL PEARLS

1. During quiet breathing, expiration results from passive recoil of the thoracic and abdominal wall.
2. In spinal cord injured persons with injuries below C4, there is a greater compromise of expiratory function than inspiratory function and inspiration improves greater than expiration over time.
3. Weakness or paralysis of internal intercostal muscles and abdominal muscles results in decreased ability to clear airway secretions, which contributes to increased risk of mucus plugging, atelectasis, and respiratory infection.

QUESTIONS

1. What is the primary muscle of inspiration and its innervation?
2. Why does an abdominal binder improve inspiratory function in the spinal cord injured patient?
3. How does respiratory muscle weakness contribute to chronic alveolar hypoventilation and list four symptoms.
4. How do the abdominal muscles contribute to both expiration and inspiration?
5. Name four accessory muscles of inspiration and their innervation.
6. How is a manually assisted cough performed?
7. Should supplemental oxygen be used to treat respiratory insufficiency due to respiratory muscle weakness?
8. What criteria would you use to begin weaning a patient with C4 ASIA A tetraplegia?
9. Define restrictive versus obstructive pulmonary dysfunction.
10. Why might weakness of upper airway muscles be a contraindication for negative pressure mechanical ventilation?

CHAPTER **10**

SWALLOWING

Richard Gray

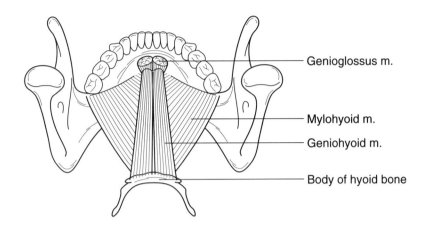

Genioglossus m.

Mylohyoid m.

Geniohyoid m.

Body of hyoid bone

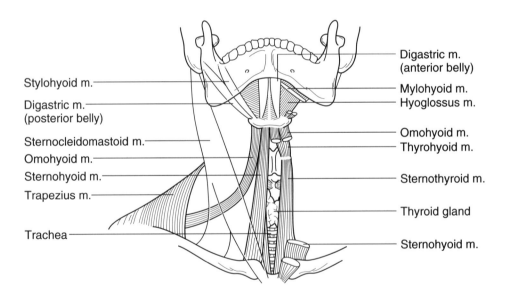

Digastric m.
(anterior belly)

Stylohyoid m.

Mylohyoid m.

Hyoglossus m.

Digastric m.
(posterior belly)

Sternocleidomastoid m.

Omohyoid m.

Thyrohyoid m.

Omohyoid m.

Sternohyoid m.

Sternothyroid m.

Trapezius m.

Thyroid gland

Trachea

Sternohyoid m.

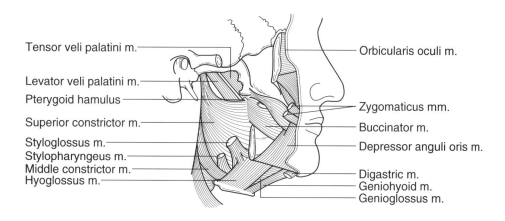

Tensor veli palatini m.
Levator veli palatini m.
Pterygoid hamulus
Superior constrictor m.
Styloglossus m.
Stylopharyngeus m.
Middle constrictor m.
Hyoglossus m.

Orbicularis oculi m.
Zygomaticus mm.
Buccinator m.
Depressor anguli oris m.
Digastric m.
Geniohyoid m.
Genioglossus m.

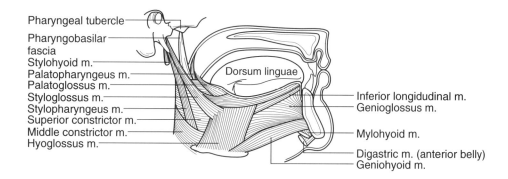

Pharyngeal tubercle
Pharyngobasilar fascia
Stylohyoid m.
Palatopharyngeus m.
Palatoglossus m.
Styloglossus m.
Stylopharyngeus m.
Superior constrictor m.
Middle constrictor m.
Hyoglossus m.

Dorsum linguae

Inferior longidudinal m.
Genioglossus m.
Mylohyoid m.
Digastric m. (anterior belly)
Geniohyoid m.

112. TENSOR VELI PALATINI (TVP)

Origin
- Fossa of the sphenoid

Insertion
- Palatine aponeurosis of the soft palate

Nerve Trigeminal (CN V)

Open Chain Actions N/A

Closed Chain Actions
- Stretches the soft palate. During the swallow the Tensor veli palatini (TVP) causes an anterior depression in the soft palate which helps to hold the bolus against the surface of the tongue.

Synergists N/A

Antagonists N/A

MUSCLE TESTING INSTRUCTIONS

See Clinical Evaluation section

CLINICAL PEARLS

1. Abnormal TVP performance may lead to poor bolus control in the oral phase. This could result in aspiration before the swallow or pocketing of material in the oral cavity.

113. LEVATOR VELI PALATINI (LVP)

Origin
- Apex of the temporal bone

Insertion
- Palatine aponeurosis of the soft palate

Nerve Vagus (CN X) and Accessory (CN XI)

Open Chain Actions N/A

Closed Chain Actions
- Raises the soft palate

Synergists N/A

Antagonists N/A

MUSCLE TESTING INSTRUCTIONS

See Clinical Evaluation section

CLINICAL PEARLS

1. Dysfunction of the LVP will result in inadequate occlusion of the nasopharynx possibly leading to nasal regurgitation of bolus material.
2. Hypernasality of speech or difficulty producing plosives ("pa," "ta," etc.) would also suggest poor closure of the nasopharynx. Detection of nasal emission of air while producing plosives may also indicate poor LVP function. This can be tested by holding a mirror under the nostrils and noting any fogging of the mirror as the patient utters repetitive plosives.

114. SALPINGOPHARYNGEUS

Origin
- Pharyngeal end of the auditory tube

Insertion
- Blends with the palatopharyngeus to insert on the posterior border of the thyroid cartilage and the pharyngeal aponeurosis

Nerve
- Pharyngeal plexus
  - Vagus(CN X)
  - Accessory(CN XI)

Open Chain Actions N/A

Closed Chain Actions
- Elevation of the larynx and pharynx

Synergists N/A

Antagonists N/A

MUSCLE TESTING INSTRUCTIONS

See Clinical Evaluation section

CLINICAL PEARLS

1. Observe for the rise of the pharynx and larynx during the pharyngeal response.

115. PALATOPHARYNGEUS

Origin
- Soft palate

Insertion
- Pharyngeal wall

Nerve
- Pharyngeal plexus
- Branch from Accessory nerve (CN XI)

Open Chain Actions N/A

Closed Chain Actions
- Occlusion of the nasopharynx
- Elevation of the pharynx
- Narrowing of the oropharynx

Synergists N/A

Antagonists N/A

MUSCLE TESTING INSTRUCTIONS

See Clinical Evaluation section

CLINICAL PEARLS

1. Observe for the rise of the pharynx during the pharyngeal phase.

116. STYLOPHARYNGEUS

Origin
- Medial aspect of the styloid process

Insertion
- Superior and inferior border of the thyroid cartilage

Nerve Glossopharyngeal (CN IX)

Open Chain Actions N/A

Closed Chain Actions Raises and dilates the wall of the pharynx

Synergists N/A

Antagonists N/A

MUSCLE TESTING INSTRUCTIONS

See Clinical Evaluation section

CLINICAL PEARLS

1. Observe for the rise of the pharynx during the pharyngeal phase.

117. SUPRAHYOID MUSCLES

- *GENIOHYOID*
- *MYLOHYOID*
- *STYLOHYOID*
- *DIGASTRIC*

Origin
- Geniohyoid: spine of the mandible
- Mylohyoid: inner surface of the mandible
- Stylohyoid: styloid process of the temporal bone
- Digastric
  - Posterior belly: mastoid process of temporal bone
  - Anterior belly: lower border of mandible

Insertion
- Geniohyoid: hyoid bone
- Mylohyoid: hyoid bone
- Stylohyoid: hyoid bone
- Digastric: a combined intermediate tendon ultimately attaching to the hyoid bone

Nerve
- Geniohyoid: hypoglossal (CN XII)
- Mylohyoid: trigeminal (CN V)
- Stylohyoid: facial (CN VII)
- Digastric: trigeminal (CN V); variably from the facial (CN VII)

Open Chain Actions N/A

Closed Chain Actions Elevation of the hyoid during the swallow. The contraction of the mylohyoid [117] also bulges the base of the tongue into the oropharynx.

Synergists N/A

Antagonists Infrahyoid muscles

MUSCLE TESTING INSTRUCTIONS

See Clinical Evaluation section

CLINICAL PEARLS

1. The tester should observe for elevation of the hyoid bone.

118. TONGUE: INTRINSIC MUSCLES

Origin
- Superior longitudinal: submucous fibrous tissue near the epiglottis and the median lingual septum
- Inferior longitudinal: lingual root
- Transverse: submucus fibrous tissue near the lingual margin
- Vertical: dorsal surface of the tongue

Insertion
- Superior longitudinal: lingual margins
- Inferior longitudinal: apex of the tongue
- Transverse: median fibrous septum
- Vertical: ventral surface of the tongue

Nerve Hypoglossal (CN XII)

Open Chain Actions

SOLO ACTIONS
- Superior longitudinal: shortens tongue, raises apex and sides of tongue
- Inferior longitudinal: shortens tongue, pulls apex downwards
- Transverse: narrows and elongates the tongue
- Vertical: flattens and widens the tongue

COMBINED ACTION The combined action of these muscles provides the tongue with very precise and highly variable mobility.

Closed Chain Actions N/A

Synergists N/A

Antagonists N/A

MUSCLE TESTING INSTRUCTIONS

Patient
Seated, facing the tester

Tester
The tester observes the following tongue movements

Test
"Stick out your tongue and then put it back in. Curve your tongue up on the sides and then curve it down."

CLINICAL PEARLS

1. Some of these actions may be difficult for the patient to "perform" on command but may be observable in transition.
2. These movements may be limited when a patient has ankyloglossia (lingua frenata). This is often colloquially referred to as being "tongue-tied."

119. TONGUE (EXTRINSIC MUSCLES)

- *HYOGLOSSUS*
- *GENIOGLOSSUS*
- *STYLOGLOSSUS*
- *PALATOGLOSSUS*

Origin
- Hyoglossus: greater cornu of the hyoid
- Genioglossus: upper genial tubercle of the mandible
- Styloglossus: anterior and lateral border of the styloid process
- Palatoglossus: anterior surface of the soft palate

Insertion
- Hyoglossus: sides of the tongue
- Genioglossus: ventral surface of the tongue
- Styloglossus: sides of the tongue
- Palatoglossus: dorsum and sides of the tongue

Nerve
- Hypoglossus: hypoglossal (CN XII)
- Genioglossus: hypoglossal (CN XII)
- Styloglossus: hypoglossal (CN XII)
- Palatoglossus: glossopharyngeal (CN IX), Vagus (CN XI)

Open Chain Actions
SOLO ACTIONS
- Hypoglossus: tongue depression
- Genioglossus: protrusion and depression of the tongue
- Styloglossus: draws tongue up and backwards
- Palatoglossus: narrows and elevates the posterior tongue

COMBINED ACTION

The combined action of these muscles gives the tongue its very precise and highly variable mobility.

Closed Chain Actions N/A

Synergists N/A

Antagonists N/A

MUSCLE TESTING INSTRUCTIONS

Patient
Seated, facing the tester

Tester
The tester is seated and observes the following tongue movements

Test
"Stick out your tongue. Lift up your tongue. Push down your tongue. Stick your tongue back. Raise the back of your tongue."

CLINICAL PEARLS

N/A

120. PHARYNGEAL CONSTRICTORS

Origin
- Inferior constrictor
  - Cricoid cartilage
  - Thyroid lamina
  - Tendinous band from the inferior thyroid tubercle to the cricoid cartilage
- Middle constrictor
  - Hyoid bone
  - Stylohyoid ligament
- Superior constrictor
  - Pterygoid
  - Mandible

Insertion Common insertion into the median pharyngeal raphe

Nerve Pharyngeal plexus

Open Chain Actions
SOLO ACTION N/A

COMBINED ACTION The constrictors provide a peristaltic motion in the pharynx. One part of the inferior constrictor provides a sphincteric action at the pharyngeal-esophageal juncture.

Closed Chain Actions N/A

Synergists N/A

Antagonists N/A

MUSCLE TESTING INSTRUCTIONS

This muscle is NOT easily accessible to clinical testing.

CLINICAL PEARLS

N/A

121. INFRAHYOID MUSCLES

- *STERNOHYOID*
- *STERNOTHYROID*
- *OMOHYOID*
- *THYROHYOID*)

Origin
- Sternhyoid
  - Medial clavicle
  - Posterior sternoclavicular ligament
  - Upper posterior manubrium sterni
- Sternothyroid
  - Posterior manubrium
  - Posterior edge of first costal cartilage
- Omohyoid
  - Upper scapular border
  - Superior transverse scapular ligament
- Thyrohyoid
  - Oblique line of the thyroid lamina

Insertion
- Sternohyoid: inferior border of the hyoid
- Sternothyroid: oblique line of the thyroid lamina
- Omohyoid: Hyoid
- Thyrohyoid: greater cornu of the hyoid

Nerve
- Sternohyoid: Ansa cervicalis
- Sternothyroid: Ansa cervicalis
- Omohyoid: Superior ramus of ansa cervicalis and ansa cervicalis
- Thyrohyoid: Hypoglossal

Open Chain Actions N/A

Closed Chain Actions
- Sternothyroid: Depression of larynx
- Sternohyoid: Depression of the hyoid
- Omohyoid: Depression of the hyoid
- Thyrohyoid: Depression of the hyoid

Synergists N/A

Antagonists Suprahyoid muscles

MUSCLE TESTING INSTRUCTIONS

See Clinical Evaluation section

CLINICAL PEARLS

1. The tester should observe for the fall of the hyoid and larynx after the swallow.

PHYSIOLOGY OF SWALLOWING

The three-stage system proposed by Logeman provides a useful conceptual framework for considering the process of swallowing:

- *Preoral Phase:* This phase begins with the introduction of material into the oral cavity and consists of those activities which lead to the formation of a consistent bolus, that is, mastication of solids, gathering and controlling semisolid and liquid materials. Actions of the tongue, masseter, labial constrictor, and buccal muscles all play a role. The preoral stage ends with the positioning of the formed bolus against the anterior hard palate.
- *Oral Phase:* This stage involves the transport of the bolus from the anterior hold position to the back of the oral cavity. Propulsion and control of the bolus is largely dependent on the action of the tongue with some assistance from the buccal musculature and soft palate in maintaining control. This phase ends with the stimulation of the pharyngeal response as the bolus passes the faucial pillars.
- *Pharyngeal Phase:* Stimulation of the pharyngeal response results in an involuntary sequence of actions. The soft palate is elevated and approximated to the posterior pharyngeal wall to occlude the nasopharynx. The hyoid bone is elevated. The pharynx and larynx are drawn up behind the hyoid. The epiglottis inverts to occlude the opening to the trachea. Pharyngeal peristalsis and constriction is initiated. The cricopharyngeus relaxes to open the pharyngeal-esophageal junction and allows the bolus to enter the esophagus.

While some overlap occurs for actions between stages and some disagreement exists for the timing of individual events (some would place the elevation of the hyoid in the oral stage, while others as an early part of the pharyngeal), this system serves as a useful framework for considering and categorizing various forms of dysphagia.

CATEGORIZATION OF SWALLOWING DISORDERS

The primary consequences of dysphagia can be categorized as:

- Poor oral intake
- Aspiration: Can be further subdivided as:
    - *Aspiration before the swallow:* Failure to form/maintain a consistent bolus during the preoral or oral phases may result in small quantities of bolus material entering into the pharynx without stimulating a pharyngeal response, thereby allowing material to fall into the open airway. This can result from dysfunction of the oral or lingual muscles or may be secondary to decreased oral sensation.
    - *Aspiration during the swallow:* If the pharyngeal response is inadequate or uncoordinated there may be inadequate closure of the airway during the swallow, again allowing bolus material to enter the airway.
    - *Aspiration after the swallow:* An inadequate/uncoordinated pharyngeal response may lead to material becoming trapped/pooled in the vallecula or piriform sinuses. When the pharyngeal response relaxes and the airway reopens this material may dislodge and fall into the open airway. A similar result may occur if material has become lodged in the oral cavity due to poor bolus formation or control. When this occurs, material usually lodges in the sulcus between the cheek and gums. If this material dislodges and enters the pharynx without stimulating another pharyngeal response, it can again result in material entering the airway.

CLINICAL EVALUATION

While the "gold standard" for the diagnosis and categorization of dysphagia involves the use of radiologic studies such as the modified barium swallow, much can be learned from the clinical examination. Although this text is primarily concerned with the physical examination, a brief mention of the important aspects of the history will be given as this is crucial in identifying individuals with swallowing problems.

History

While a history of coughing or choking associated with eating or drinking may be considered the "classical" presentation for patients with dysphagia, it should be remembered that large numbers of patients with swallowing disorders will experience silent aspiration with little or no clinical signs. Therefore, it is important to be alert for reports of more subtle changes. Patients may report or be reported to have changes in eating habits, such as avoiding certain consistencies, taking longer to eat than expected, weight loss, abnormal lab studies such as low albumin or pre-albumin. Reports of "drooling" and nasal regurgitation not only indicate that there are oral problems directly related to these, but also should raise questions concerning oral dysfunction that could lead to poor bolus formation and control which may lead to aspiration. While patient reports of food "sticking" in the throat are often difficult to evaluate, such symptoms can result from pooling in the piriform sinuses or vallecula. A history of recurrent pnuemonia may also indicate possible dysphagia.

Physical Examination

The physical examination can be divided into two sections, direct and functional testing.

- *DIRECT TESTING*

The oral cavity should be inspected for any obvious lesions. Any dryness of the oral mucosa should be noted (this may indicate dehydration as well as interfere with swallowing). The teeth should be inspected including the fit of dentures, as this may affect the patient's ability to handle solids. Strength of the masseter muscles and adequacy of labial closure may be tested by direct challenge. Lingual function can be tested by asking the patient to stick out the tongue. Weakness of the intrinsic muscles will result in the tongue's deviation to the side of the weakness. The patient should be asked to touch the front of the hard palate with the tip of the tongue and then sweep it backward along the palate. The patient should also be asked to sweep the sulcii between the cheek and the gum. A final test of lingual function should be to raise the back of the tongue to the roof of the mouth. This can be facilitated by asking the patient to make a "k" sound. Pharyngeal sensitivity can be tested by eliciting the "gag reflex." It is important to remember, however, that an absent gag does not mean that there is a swallowing problem and that a positive gag does not ensure the safety of the swallow.

While not strictly a "direct" assessment of the swallow, information can be obtained by listening to and analyzing a patient's speech. The presence of dysarthria may indicate oral motor problems that could affect the swallow. The presence of hypernasality or difficulty producing plosive sounds such as "pa" or "ta" may indicate inadequate closure of the nasopharynx. The escape of air from the nose, indicated by fogging of a mirror held under the nostrils, while making plosive sounds, would also indicate poor closure of the nasopharynx by the soft palate

- *FUNCTIONAL TESTING*

Test swallows are commonly carried out using ten cc (two teaspoons) boluses. Larger boluses of 30 ccs can also be used with liquids. In general, four consistencies of bolus are used:

- Thin liquids (a consistency similar to water)
- Thick liquids (a consistency similar to a milk shake)
- Paste (a consistency similar to pudding)
- Solid (a consistency similar to a cookie)

The exact sequence of testing can vary, though.

The bolus can be placed in the mouth by either the patient or the tester, and the patient is instructed to swallow. The tester should watch for any loss of material from the mouth during the oral and preoral phases. In cases where oral dysfunction limits the ability to form, control, or transport the bolus, one may note very labored motions of the tongue, tipping of the head, etc. Any coughing or choking noted before the initiation of the pharyngeal response (see below) suggests aspiration occurring before the swallow.

With the initiation of the pharyngeal response, the rise of the hyoid and larynx will be noted. Visual observation can be supplemented by gently placing the hand over the anterior aspect of the neck to feel the rise of these landmarks. Completion of the pharyngeal response will be signaled by the lowering of these structures to their resting position. The presence of coughing or choking during this phase suggests aspiration occurring during the swallow.

Once the pharyngeal phase has subsided the patient should be observed for any signs of coughing or choking which may indicate aspiration after the swallow from pooled material in either the oral cavity or pharynx, that is, aspiration after the swallow. Some patients may also demonstrate a second pharyngeal response after the initial swallow without the introduction of another bolus. This suggests that there may be material pooled in the pharynx that the patient is attempting to clear.

Immediately after completing a swallow, a patient should be asked to vocalize. In some cases where aspiration has occurred, particularly with a liquid bolus, a "wet" or "gurgling" quality to the voice may be noted. Other investigators have advocated the use of a stethoscope placed over the larynx to detect the sound of material entering the airway. The oral cavity should also be checked after each swallow to determine if any material has become trapped.

In all test swallows, there is obviously a risk of aspiration occurring.

While the clinical examination can provide valuable information, it is not a substitute for studies such as the modified barium swallow or the fiberoptic-endoscopic evaluation of the swallow (FEES) which provide far more detailed information.

QUESTIONS

1. List symptoms that may indicate the presence of a swallowing problem.
2. Describe "silent aspiration."
3. What impairments could lead to "aspiration before the swallow"?
4. What impairments could lead to "aspiration during the swallow"?
5. What impairments could lead to "aspiration after the swallow"?
6. What symptoms and/or clinical exam findings would be present with "aspiration before the swallow"?
7. What symptoms and/or clinical exam findings would be present with "aspiration during the swallow"?
8. What symptoms and/or clinical exam findings would be present with "aspiration after the swallow"?
9. What bolus sizes are most commonly used for "test swallows"?
10. What bolus consistencies are most commonly used for "test swallows"?

CHAPTER 11

MANUAL MUSCLE TESTING OF THE PEDIATRIC PATIENT

Pamela E. Wilson and Dennis J. Matthews

Muscle testing the pediatric patient is different from the technique used in adult practice. In testing children, it is essential to have an understanding of normal growth and development. In the very young child, the use of reflexes will assist in the evaluation process. In the older child, the use of developmental tasks will help to assess muscle activity. Pediatric muscle testing will be presented here by dividing the exam into three age and developmental categories:

- Infants: Birth through 12 months
- Toddler: 12 months through 24 months
- Preschooler: 24 months through 48 months

(Children over 4 years of age can be more formally tested.)

List of Key Early Reflexes

Reflex	Emergence	Disappearance
Moro	Birth	5 to 6 months
Palmar grasp	Birth	3 months
Plantar grasp	Birth	12 months
Placing	Birth	12 months
Protective: lateral	6 to 9 months	Persists
Protective: parachute	9 months	Persists

List of Key Developmental Milestones

Age	Activity
Birth	Flexion of limbs
	Ventral suspension, head in line with body
3 months	Head control midline
	Reaches for objects
	Head upright in prone
6 months	Sits with balance from hands
	Can bear weight on legs
	Transfers objects hand to hand

9 months	Sits independently
	Pulls to stand
	Crawling and cruising
	Pincer grasp
12 months	Walking alone
18 months	Creeps up stairs
	Throws a ball
24 months	Runs
	Walks up and down steps
	Kicks a ball
30 months	Jumps
36 months	Stands on one foot momentarily
	Tandem walking wobbly
48 months	Hops on one foot
	Throws a ball overhand
60 months	Skips

THE MUSCULOSKELETAL EXAM

Key Points
- Observation is essential in evaluating children.
- The exam begins as soon as the parents and child enter the room.
- Examine the infant and toddler in the parent's lap.
- The parents may need to be active participants in the exam.
- In planning the exam, move from observation to hands-on examination.
- Use normal development to help plan the exam.

THE INFANT EXAM
- Remember, development is the acquisition of new skills.
- Development is from proximal to distal and from rostral to caudal.
- Reflexes and positioning are key to the exam.

1. Observation
- Look at head position and head control.
- Observe how the child sits, and evaluate trunk control.
- Observe the upper extremities for position and movement.
- Observe the older child in standing.
- Look for any asymmetry in movement.

2. Evaluation
SUPINE
- In supine position young infants should have the arms and legs in flexion. By straightening the limb, the child will recoil back into this position (Fig. 11-1).
- Check plantar and palmar reflexes (finger and toe flexors).
- Pull the infant upward by the hands to evaluate head control, elbow flexion, and shoulder stabilization. At 5 to 6 months, the child will lift the head before the shoulders move (Fig. 11-2).

PRONE
- Place the child prone. An infant should be able to turn the head side to side. A 3-month-old child can lift the head and shoulders off the table. This evaluates neck extensors, upper spinal extensors, and elbow extensors (Fig. 11-3).

VERTICAL
- Hold the child vertical to evaluate proximal shoulder muscles and shoulder stabilizers (Fig. 11-4).

- With the child upright, tilt side to side to watch for the head righting reflex which shows lateral neck flexion.
- With child upright, place the dorsum of the foot against a solid surface to evaluate placing response (hip and knee flexion).
- Check the parachute protective response in a child who is 9 months or older (Fig. 11-5)

HORIZONTAL

- Hold the child horizontal, the Landau reflex will cause neck extension, spine extension, and hip extension (Fig. 11-6).
- Stroking the spine will cause a movement toward the side stimulated. This is a Galant reflex.
- This is a good place to do a Moro reflex as you are already manipulating the child. While holding the child supine on the arm, suddenly drop the head about 30 degrees and watch for abduction of the shoulder and extension of the elbow and fingers, followed by adduction of the shoulder and flexion of the elbow.

SITTING

- Evaluate the child in the sitting position. How much support is needed? Can the child do this independently? Are the lateral protective reflexes present (shift the child to the side and the arm should extend) (Fig. 11-7)?
- Give the child a toy to assess hand and shoulder function. Have the child reach for it overhead to evaluate shoulder and elbow extension. If the toy is placed laterally, it evaluates shoulder abduction.
- Place a small object on the table and evaluate the grasp as child picks it up (raking or pincer) (Fig. 11-8).

FLOOR PLAY

- Place the child on a carpeted floor or mat and, if appropriate, observe transition from supine to sit. Try to encourage crawling by using a toy.

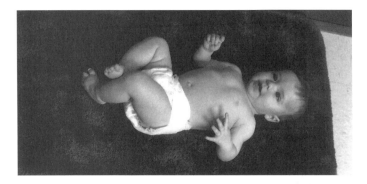

Figure 11-1

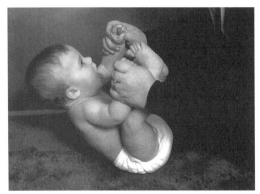

Figure 11-2

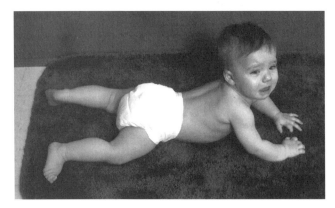

Figure 11-3

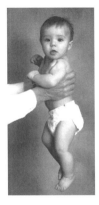

Figure 11-4

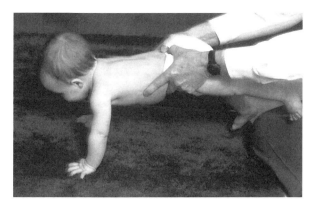

Figure 11-5

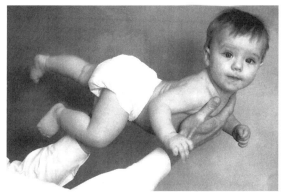

Figure 11-6

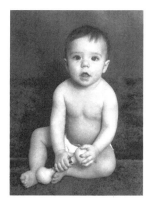

Figure 11-7

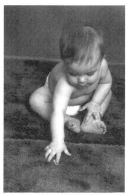

Figure 11-8

THE TODDLER EXAM
- This can be a very challenging exam. Parental assistance is invaluable.
- Get as much information as possible to get muscle information from a child who is resisting the exam.
- Remember normal development.
- Have toys available.

1. Observation
- Watch the family enter the room. If the child is being carried, look at the head and spine stability, position of the arms and legs, and general movement patterns. If the child can walk, evaluate the base of support, gait pattern, balance, and postural responses, along with posture.

2. Evaluation
SITTING ON THE TABLE OR PARENT'S LAP
- Evaluate the upper extremity function by having the child grasp a toy directly in front, overhead, and to the side. This will demonstrate antigravity shoulder flexion and abduction. As the child looks up, this will evaluate neck extension.
- Adding a second toy will encourage the child to transfer objects to the opposite hand (either shoulder internal rotation or shoulder adduction along with wrist and finger extension). Pronation can be demonstrated by having the child give back the toy to the examiner or parent.
- Check the lateral protective reflexes while sitting.
- In this position, the lower extremities can be screened for ankle dorsiflexion by stroking the foot. Knee extension can be examined by trying to get the child to kick at an object.
- Children will often abduct and adduct the hips in sitting. Be observant of this.

FLOOR EXAM
- Place the child supine and watch transition into sit (a child cannot sit without rolling until 3 years). Muscles required for this activity include those of the trunk, pelvis, shoulder, wrist, and fingers. If a child cannot do this or adds other movements, start thinking weakness. Check the neck flexors formally by having the child pull to sit.
- Have the child stand up. Watch the trunk and lower extremities.
- Ask the child to walk and run around the room. If possible, have the child walk up stairs (hip extension, hip abduction, knee flexion, and ankle dorsiflexion are all assessed by these activities).
- Have a child kick a ball (hip flexion) and throw the ball at the parent (shoulder flexion and elbow extension).

THE PRESCHOOL EXAM
- Generally this group is more cooperative.
- Testing is still by muscle groups unless there is a need to isolate a particular muscle.
- Remember the developmental milestones.

1. Observation
- Watch the child walk into the room and watch all subsequent activities.

2. Evaluation
SITTING ON THE EXAM TABLE
- Look at the sitting posture.
- Check the neck flexors by having the child look at the belly button and applying resistance to the forehead. Then, check the neck extensors by having the child look at the ceiling and applying resistance to the back of the head.

- To test shoulder strength, have the child hold his or her arms out like a bird in abduction and apply resistance or use the previous technique of having him or her grab an object overhead (this also evaluates elbow extension).
- To check elbow flexion, have the child grab an ear and hold it while the examiner applies resistance.
- Have the child hold the arms against the body while the examiner tries to pull these away from the body (shoulder adduction).
- In testing the lower extremities, have the child kick the leg forward (knee extension).

LYING ON THE EXAM TABLE
- Have the child lift the leg off the table (hip flexors).
- Have him or her come to a sitting position with the examiner holding his or her hands (neck flexors, trunk flexors). If there is a suspicion of neck flexor weakness, hang the child's head, supported over the end of the table, and then slowly remove the support. Feel for the movement of the head upward.

FLOOR EXAM
- Watch the walking pattern of the child. Look for a Trendelenburg style or asymmetry of gait.
- Have the child run down the hallway.
- Have the child jump.
- Have the child stand on one foot (3 years).
- Walk on tiptoes (3 years).
- Try tandem walking (3 years).
- Have the child hop on one foot (4 years).
- Have the child skip (5 years).
- Lay the child on the floor supine and have him or her stand up quickly, not using assistance to get up. Watch for a Gower's maneuver, using the upper extremities to climb up the legs, to get upright.
- Evaluate the child going up and down stairs.

SUMMARY

Muscle testing children can easily be accomplished by knowing normal development and growth. Using these as tools, the different muscle groups can be evaluated in reflexive and functional patterns. Observation and flexibility are key to the exam.

QUESTIONS

1. At what age should a child be sitting independently?
2. Discuss the approach to muscle testing an infant.
3. Discuss the approach to muscle testing a toddler.
4. Discuss the approach to muscle testing a preschooler.
5. At what age range should a child be walking independently?
6. Discuss the development of grasp techniques.

7. When an infant is held vertically, what aspects of the exam should you observe?
8. In supine, what aspects of the exam should be observed?
9. Discuss how you would engage a nonparticipating child in the examination.
10. How do you evaluate posture and postural reflexes in a child?

APPENDICES

APPENDIX 1: ALPHABETICAL LIST OF MUSCLES

- Abdominals
  - External Abdominal Oblique (T5-L1) [83]
  - Internal Abdominal Oblique (T5-L1) [84]
  - Rectus Abdominis (T5-T12) [82]
  - Quadratus Lumborum (T12-L1) [85]
- Abductor Digiti Minimi (Foot) (S1-2) [81]
- Abductor Digiti Minimi (Hand) (C8-T1) [44]
- Abductor Hallucis (S1-2) [77]
- Abductor Pollicis Brevis (C7-T1) [39]
- Abductor Pollicis Longus (C6-8) [30]
- Adductor Brevis and Longus (L2-4) [56]
- Adductor Magnus (L2-S1) [57]
- Adductor Pollicis (C8-T1) [46]
- Anterior Deltoid (C5-6) [12]
- Anterior Scalenus (Ventral rami C3-8) [108]
- Anterior Tibialis (L4-S1) [66]
- Biceps Brachii (C5-6) [20]
- Biceps Femoris (Short and Long Heads)
  (L5-S2) [63]
- Brachialis (C5-7) [21]
- Brachioradialis (C5-6) [23]
- Buccinator (CNVII) [99]
- Coracobrachialis (C5-7) [19]
- Deltoid
  - Anterior Deltoid (C5-6) [12]
  - Middle Deltoid (C5-6) [13]
  - Posterior Deltoid (C5-6) [14]
- Depressor Anguli Oris (CNVII) [100]
- Diaphragm (C3-5) [109]
- Digastric (CNV) [117]
- Dorsal Interossei (Foot) (S1-2) [80]
- Dorsal Interossei (Hand) (C8-T1) [48]
- Extensor Carpi Radialis Longus and Brevis
  (C6-7) [25]
- Extensor Carpi Ulnaris (C6-8) [27]
- Extensor Digitorum Brevis (L5-S1) [70]
- Extensor Digitorum Communis (C6-8) [26]
- Extensor Digitorum Longus (L4-S1) [67]
- Extensor Hallucis Longus (L5-S1) [68]
- Extensor Indicis (C6-8) [28]

- Extensor Pollicis Brevis (C6-8) [31]
- Extensor Pollicis Longus (C6-8) [29]
- External Abdominal Oblique (T5-L1) [83]
- External Intercostals (T1-11) [110]
- Flexor Carpi Radialis (C6-8) [33]
- Flexor Carpi Ulnaris (C8-T1) [50]
- Flexor Digiti Minimi (C8-T1) [45]
- Flexor Digitorum Longus (L5-S1) [74]
- Flexor Digitorum Profundus (C7-T1) [37]
- Flexor Digitorum Superficialis (C7-T1) [35]
- Flexor Hallucis Longus (L5-S2) [75]
- Flexor Pollicis Brevis: Deep and Superficial Heads
  (C7-T1) [41]
- Flexor Pollicis Longus (C7-T1) [36]
- Frontalis (CNVII) [92]
- Gastrocnemius (L5-S2) [72]
- Genioglossus (CNXII) [119]
- Geniohyoid (CNXII) [117]
- Gluteus Maximus (L5-S2) [52]
- Gluteus Medius (L4-S1) [53]
- Gluteus Minimus (L4-S1) [54]
- Gracilis (L2-4) [59]
- Hip Rotators (Piriformis) (S1-2) [60]
- Hyoglossus (CNXII) [119]
- Iliocostalis Cervicis, Thoracis, and Lumborum
  [86]
- Iliopsoas (L2-4) [51]
- Infrahyoid Muscles [121]
  - Omohyoid (Superior Ramus of Ansa Cervicalis and
    Ansa Cervicalis)
  - Sternohyoid (Ansa Cervicalis)
  - Sternothyroid (Ansa Cervicalis)
  - Thyrohyoid (CNX11)
- Infraspinatus (C5-6) [18]
- Internal Abdominal Oblique (T5-L1) [84]
- Internal Intercostals (T1-11) [111]
- Lateral and Medial Pterygoids (CNV) [103]
- Latissimus Dorsi (C6-8) [7]
- Levator Palpebrae Superioris (CNIII, Sympathetic)
  [96]

- Levator Scapulae (C3-5) [5]
- Levator Veli Palatini (CNX, XI) [113]
- Longissimus Capitis, Cervicis, and Thoracis [87]
- Lower Trapezius (CNXI, C2-4) [3]
- Lumbricales (Foot) (L5-S2) [78]
- Lumbricals (Hand) (C7-T1) [42]
- Masseter (CNV) [101]
- Medial and Lateral Pterygoids (CNV) [103]
- Middle Deltoid (C5-6) [13]
- Middle Scalenus (Ventral Rami C3-8) [108]
- Middle Trapezius (CNXI, C2-4) [2]
- Multifidus [90]
- Mylohyoid (CNV) [117]
- Nasalis (CNVII) [93]
- Obliquus Capitis Superior and Inferior (Dorsal Rami C1-2) [106]
- Omohyoid (Superior Ramus of Ansa Cervicalis and Ansa Cervicalis) [121]
- Opponens Digiti Minimi (C8-T1) [43]
- Opponens Pollicis (C7-T1) [40]
- Orbicularis Oculi (CNVII) [95]
- Orbicularis Oris (CNVII) [97]
- Palatoglossus (CNIX, XI) [119]
- Palatopharyngeus (CNXI, Pharyngeal Plexus) [115]
- Palmaris Brevis (C7-T1) [49]
- Palmar Interossei (C8-T1) [47]
- Palmaris Longus (C7-T1) [34]
- Pectineus (L2-4) [58]
- Pectoralis Major Clavicular Portion (C5-7) [9]
- Pectoralis Major Sternal Portion (C8-T1) [10]
- Pectoralis Minor (C7-T1) [11]
- Peroneii (Peroneus Longus and Brevis) (L4-S1) [71]
- Peroneus Tertius (L4-S1) [69]
- Pharyngeal Constrictors (Pharyngeal Plexus) [120]
- Piriformis [60]
- Plantar Interossei (S1-2) [79]
- Platysma / Depressor Anguli Oris (CNVII) [100]
- Popliteus (L4-S1) [65]
- Posterior Deltoid (C5-6) [14]
- Posterior Tibialis (L5-S1) [76]
- Posterior Scalenus (Ventral Rami C3-8) [108]
- Procerus (CNVII) [94]
- Pronator Quadratus (C7-T1) [38]
- Pronator Teres (C6-7) [32]
- Pterygoids (Lateral and Medial) (CNV) [103]
- Quadratus Lumborum (T12-L1) [85]
- Quadriceps (Rectus Femoris, Vastus Lateralis, Medialis, and Intermedius) (L2-4) [62]
- Rectus Abdominis (T5-T12) [82]
- Rectus Capitis Posterior Major and Minor (Dorsal Rami C1-2) [105]
- Rectus Femoris (L2-4) [62]
- Rhomboid Major and Minor (C5) [4]

- Rotator Cuff Muscles
  - Infraspinatus (C5-6) [18]
  - Subscapularis (C5-6) [16]
  - Supraspinatus (C5-6) [17]
  - Teres Minor (C5-6) [15]
- Rotatores [91]
- Salpingopharyngeus (CNX, XI) [114]
- Sartorius (L2-4) [61]
- Scalenus (Anterior, Medius and Posterior) (Ventral Rami C3-8) [108]
- Semispinalis Capitis and Cervicis [89]
- Semitendinosus and Semimembranosus (L5-S2) [64]
- Serratus Anterior (C5-7) [6]
- Soleus (L5-S2) [73]
- Spinalis Capitis, Cervicis, and Thoracis [88]
- Splenius Capitis and Cervicis (Dorsal Rami C3-8) [104]
- Sternocleidomastoid (CNXI, C2-3) [107]
- Sternohyoid (Ansa Cervicalis) [121]
- Sternothyroid (Ansa Cervicalis) [121]
- Styloglossus (CNXII) [119]
- Stylohyoid (CNVII) [117]
- Stylopharyngeus (CNIX) [116]
- Subscapularis (C5-6) [16]
- Supinator (C5-6) [24]
- Suprahyoid Muscles [117]
  - Digastric (CNV)
  - Geniohyoid (CNXII)
  - Mylohyoid (CNV)
  - Stylohyoid (CNVII)
- Supraspinatus (C5-6) [17]
- Temporalis (CNV) [102]
- Tensor Fascia Lata (L4-S1) [55]
- Tensor Veli Palatini (CNV) [112]
- Teres Major (C5-6) [8]
- Teres Minor (C5-6) [15]
- Thyrohyoid (CNXII) [121]
- Tibialis Anterior (L4-S1) [66]
- Tibialis Posterior (L5-S1) [76]
- Trapezius
  - Lower Trapezius (CNXI, C2-4) [3]
  - Middle Trapezius (CNXI, C2-4) [2]
  - Upper Trapezius (CNXI, C2-4) [1]
- Triceps Brachii and Anconeus (C6-8) [22]
- Tongue (CNXII) [118]
- Tongue Extrinsic Muscles [119]
  - Genioglossus (CNXII)
  - Hyoglossus (CNXII)
  - Palatoglossus (CNIX, XI)
  - Styloglossus (CNXII)
- Upper Trapezius (CNXI, C2-4) [1]
- Vastus Intermedius (L2-4) [62]
- Vastus Lateralis (L2-4) [62]
- Vastus Medialis (L2-4) [62]
- Zygomaticus Major and Minor (CNVII) [98]

APPENDIX 2: LIST OF MUSCLES BY NUMBER

1. Upper Trapezius (CNXI, C2-4)
2. Middle Trapezius (CNXI, C2-4)
3. Lower Trapezius (CNXI, C2-4)
4. Rhomboid Major and Minor (C5)
5. Levator Scapulae (C3-5)
6. Serratus Anterior (C5-7)
7. Latissimus Dorsi (C6-8)
8. Teres Major (C5-6)
9. Pectoralis Major Clavicular Portion (C5-7)
10. Pectoralis Major Sternal Portion (C8-T1)
11. Pectoralis Minor (C7-T1)
12. Anterior Deltoid (C5-6)
13. Middle Deltoid (C5-6)
14. Posterior Deltoid (C5-6)
15. Teres Minor (C5-6)
16. Subscapularis (C5-6)
17. Supraspinatus (C5-6)
18. Infraspinatus (C5-6)
19. Coracobrachialis (C5-7)
20. Biceps Brachii (C5-6)
21. Brachialis (C5-7)
22. Triceps Brachii and Anconeus (C6-8)
23. Brachioradialis (C5-6)
24. Supinator (C5-6)
25. Extensor Carpi Radialis Longus and Brevis (C6-7)
26. Extensor Digitorum Communis (C6-8)
27. Extensor Carpi Ulnaris (C6-8)
28. Extensor Indicis (C6-8)
29. Extensor Pollicis Longus (C6-8)
30. Abductor Pollicis Longus (C6-8)
31. Extensor Pollicis Brevis (C6-8)
32. Pronator Teres (C6-7)
33. Flexor Carpi Radialis (C6-8)
34. Palmaris Longus (C7-T1)
35. Flexor Digitorum Superficialis (C7-T1)
36. Flexor Pollicis Longus (C7-T1)
37. Flexor Digitorum Profundus (C7-T1)
38. Pronator Quadratus (C7-T1)
39. Abductor Pollicis Brevis (C7-T1)
40. Opponens Pollicis (C7-T1)
41. Flexor Pollicis Brevis: Deep and Superficial Heads (C7-T1)
42. Lumbricals (C7-T1)
43. Opponens Digiti Minimi (C8-T1)
44. Abductor Digiti Minimi (C8-T1)
45. Flexor Digiti Minimi (C8-T1)
46. Adductor Pollicis (C8-T1)
47. Palmar Interossei (C8-T1)
48. Dorsal Interossei (C8-T1)
49. Palmaris Brevis (C7-T1)
50. Flexor Carpi Ulnaris (C8-T1)
51. Iliopsoas (L2-4)
52. Gluteus Maximus (L5-S2)
53. Gluteus Medius (L4-S1)
54. Gluteus Minimus (L4-S1)
55. Tensor Fascia Lata (L4-S1)
56. Adductor Brevis and Longus (L2-4)
57. Adductor Magnus (L2-S1)
58. Pectineus (L2-4)
59. Gracilis (L2-4)
60. Hip Rotators (Piriformis) (S1-2)
61. Sartorius (L2-4)
62. Quadriceps (Rectus Femoris, Vastus Lateralis, Medialis, and Intermedius) (L2-4)
63. Biceps Femoris (Short and Long Heads) (L5-S2)
64. Semitendinosus and Semimembranosus (L5-S2)
65. Popliteus (L4-S1)
66. Tibialis Anterior (L4-S1)
67. Extensor Digitorum Longus (L4-S1)
68. Extensor Hallucis Longus (L5-S1)
69. Peroneus Tertius (L4-S1)
70. Extensor Digitorum Brevis (L5-S1)
71. Peroneii (Peroneus Longus and Brevis) (L4-S1)
72. Gastrocnemius (L5-S2)
73. Soleus (L5-S2)
74. Flexor Digitorum Longus (L5-S1)
75. Flexor Hallucis Longus (L5-S2)
76. Tibialis Posterior (L5-S1)
77. Abductor Hallucis (S1-2)
78. Lumbricales (L5-S2)
79. Plantar Interossei (S1-2)
80. Dorsal Interossei (S1-2)
81. Abductor Digiti Minimi (S1-2)
82. Rectus Abdominis (T5-T12)
83. External Abdominal Oblique (T5-L1)
84. Internal Abdominal Oblique (T5-L1)
85. Quadratus Lumborum (T12-L1)
86. Iliocostalis Cervicis, Thoracis, and Lumborum
87. Longissimus Capitis, Cervicis, and Thoracis
88. Spinalis Capitis, Cervicis, and Thoracis
89. Semispinalis Capitis and Cervicis
90. Multifidus
91. Rotatores
92. Frontalis (CNVII)
93. Nasalis (CNVII)
94. Procerus (CNVII)
95. Orbicularis Oculi (CNVII)
96. Levator Palpebrae Superioris (CNIII, Sympathetic)
97. Orbicularis Oris (CNVII)
98. Zygomaticus Major and Minor (CNVII)
99. Buccinator (CNVII)
100. Platysma / Depressor Anguli Oris (CNVII)
101. Masseter (CNV)
102. Temporalis (CNV)
103. Medial and Lateral Pterygoids (CNV)

104. Splenius Capitis and Cervicis (Dorsal Rami C3-8)
105. Rectus Capitis Posterior Major and Minor (Dorsal Rami C1-2)
106. Obliquus Capitis Superior and Inferior (Dorsal Rami C1-2)
107. Sternocleidomastoid (CNXI, C2-3)
108. Scalenus (Anterior, Medius, and Posterior) (Ventral Rami C3-8)
109. Diaphragm (C3-5)
110. External Intercostals (T1-11)
111. Internal Intercostals (T1-11)
112. Tensor Veli Palatini (CNV)
113. Levator Veli Palatini (CNX, XI)
114. Salpingopharyngeus (CNX, XI)

115. Palatopharyngeus (CNXI, Pharyngeal Plexus)
116. Stylopharyngeus (CNIX)
117. Suprahyoid Muscles: Geniohyoid (CNXII), Mylohyoid (CNV), Stylohyoid (CNVII), Digastric (CNV)
118. Tongue (CNXII)
119. Tongue Extrinsic Muscles: Hyoglossus (CNXII), Genioglossus (CNXII), Styloglossus (CNXII), Palatoglossus (CNIX, XI)
120. Pharyngeal Constrictors (Pharyngeal Plexus)
121. Infrahyoid Muscles: Sternohyoid (Ansa Cervicalis), Sternothyroid (Ansa Cervicalis), Omohyoid (Superior Ramus of Ansa Cervicalis and Ansa Cervicalis), Thyrohyoid (CNX11)

APPENDIX 3: INNERVATION

SPINAL ACCESSORY
1. Upper Trapezius (CNXI, C2-4)
2. Middle Trapezius (CNXI, C2-4)
3. Lower Trapezius (CNXI, C2-4)

DORSAL SCAPULAR
4. Rhomboid Major and Minor (C5)
5. Levator Scapulae (C3-5)

LONG THORACIC
6. Serratus Anterior (C5-7)

THORACODORSAL
7. Latissimus Dorsi (C6-8)

LOWER SUBSCAPULAR
8. Teres Major (C5-6)
16. Subscapularis (C5-6)

UPPER SUBSCAPULAR
16. Subscapularis (C5-6)

LATERAL PECTORAL
9. Pectoralis Major (Clavicular Portion) (C5-7)
10. Pectoralis Major (Sternal Portion) (C8-T1)

MEDIAL PECTORAL
10. Pectoralis Major (Sternal Portion) (C8-T1)
11. Pectoralis Minor (C7-T1)

AXILLARY
12. Anterior Deltoid (C5-6)
13. Middle Deltoid (C5-6)
14. Posterior Deltoid (C5-6)
15. Teres Minor (C5-6)

SUPRASCAPULAR
17. Supraspinatus (C5-6)
18. Infraspinatus (C5-6)

MUSCULOCUTANEOUS
19. Coracobrachialis (C5-7)
20. Biceps Brachii (C5-6)
21. Brachialis (C5-7)

RADIAL
21. Brachialis (C5-7)
22. Triceps Brachii and Anconeus (C6-8)
23. Brachioradialis (C5-6)
24. Supinator (C5-6)
25. Extensor Carpi Radialis Longus and Brevis (C6-7)
26. Extensor Digitorum Communis (C6-8)
27. Extensor Carpi Ulnaris (C6-8)
28. Extensor Indicis (C6-8)
29. Extensor Pollicis Longus (C6-8)
30. Abductor Pollicis Longus (C6-8)
31. Extensor Pollicis Brevis (C6-8)

MEDIAN
32. Pronator Teres (C6-7)
33. Flexor Carpi Radialis (C6-8)
34. Palmaris Longus (C7-T1)
35. Flexor Digitorum Superficialis (C7-T1)
36. Flexor Pollicis Longus (C7-T1)
37. Flexor Digitorum Profundus (C7-T1)
38. Pronator Quadratus (C7-T1)
39. Abductor Pollicis Brevis (C7-T1)
40. Opponens Pollicis (C7-T1)
41. Flexor Pollicis Brevis: Deep and Superficial Heads (C7-T1)
42. Lumbricals (C7-T1)

ULNAR
43. Opponens Digiti Minimi (C8-T1)
44. Abductor Digiti Minimi (C8-T1)
45. Flexor Digiti Minimi (C8-T1)
46. Adductor Pollicis (C8-T1)
47. Palmar Interossei (C8-T1)
48. Dorsal Interossei (C8-T1)
49. Palmaris Brevis (C7-T1)
37. Flexor Digitorum Profundus (C7-T1)
41. Flexor Pollicis Brevis: Deep and Superficial Heads (C7-T1)

42. Lumbricals (C7-T1)
50. Flexor Carpi Ulnaris (C8-T1)

FEMORAL
51. Iliopsoas (L2-4) (Iliacus Component only)
61. Sartorius (L2-4)
62. Quadriceps (Rectus Femoris, Vastus Lateralis, Medialis, and Intermedius) (L2-4)

INFERIOR GLUTEAL
52. Gluteus Maximus (L5-S2)

SUPERIOR GLUTEAL
53. Gluteus Medius (L4-S1)
54. Gluteus Minimus (L4-S1)
55. Tensor Fascia Lata (L4-S1)

OBTURATOR
56. Adductor Brevis and Longus (L2-4)
57. Adductor Magnus (L2-S1)
58. Pectineus (L2-4)
59. Gracilis (L2-4)

SACRAL PLEXUS
60. Hip Rotators (Piriformis) (S1-2)

SCIATIC (TIBIAL AND PERONEAL DIVISIONS)
63. Biceps Femoris (Short and Long Heads) (L5-S2)
64. Semitendinosus and Semimembranosus (L5-S2)
57. Adductor Magnus (L2-S1)

DEEP PERONEAL
66. Tibialis Anterior (L4-S1)
67. Extensor Digitorum Longus (L4-S1)
68. Extensor Hallucis Longus (L5-S1)
69. Peroneus Tertius (L4-S1)
70. Extensor Digitorum Brevis (L5-S1)

SUPERFICIAL PERONEAL
71. Peroneii (Peroneus Longus and Brevis) (L4-S1)

TIBIAL
72. Gastrocnemius (L5-S2)
73. Soleus (L5-S2)
74. Flexor Digitorum Longus (L5-S1)
75. Flexor Hallucis Longus (L5-S2)
76. Tibialis Posterior (L5-S1)
65. Popliteus (L4-S1)

PLANTAR NERVES
77. Abductor Hallucis (S1-2) (Medial Plantar)
78. Lumbricals (L5-S2) (Medial and Lateral Plantar)
79. Plantar Interossei (S1-2) (Lateral Plantar)
80. Dorsal Interossei (S1-2) (Lateral Plantar)
81. Abductor Digiti Minimi (S1-2) (Lateral Plantar)

SPINAL VENTRAL ROOTS
82. Rectus Abdominis (T5-T12)
83. External Oblique (T5-L1)
84. Internal Oblique (T5-L1)
85. Quadratus Lumborum (T12-L1)

SPINAL DORSAL ROOTS
86. Iliocostalis Cervicis, Thoracis, and Lumborum
87. Longissimus Capitis, Cervicis, and Thoracis
88. Spinalis Capitis, Cervicis, and Thoracis
89. Semispinalis Capitis and Cervicis
90. Multifidus
91. Rotatores

PHRENIC
109. Diaphragm (C3-5)

INTERCOSTALS
110. External Intercostals (T1-11)
111. Internal Intercostals (T1-11)
82. Rectus Abdominis (T5-T12)
83. External Oblique (T5-L1)
84. Internal Oblique (T5-L1)
85. Quadratus Lumborum (T12-L1)

CNIII
96. Levator palpebrae Superioris

CNV
101. Masseter
102. Temporalis
103. Medial and Lateral Pterygoids
112. Tensor Veli Palatini
114. Mylohyoid
117. Digastric

CNVII
92. Frontalis
93. Nasalis
94. Procerus
96. Orbicularis Oculi
97. Orbicularis Oris
98. Zygomaticus Major and Minor
99. Buccinator
100. Platysma/Depressor Anguli Oris
117. Stylohyoid

CNIX
116. Stylopharyngeus
119. Palatoglossus

CNX
113. Levator Veli Palatini
114. Salpingopharyngeus

CNXI
1. Upper Trapezius
2. Middle Trapezius
3. Lower Trapezius
107. Sternocleidomastoid
113. Levator Veli Palatini
114. Salpingopharyngeus
115. Palatopharyngeus
119. Palatoglossus

CNXII
117. Geniohyoid
118. Tongue
119. Hyoglossus
119. Genioglossus
119. Styloglossus
121. Thyrohyoid

ANSA CERVICALIS
121. Sternohyoid

121. Sternothyroid
121. Omohyoid

SYMPATHETIC
96. Levator Palpebrae Superioris

PHARYNGEAL PLEXUS
115. Palatopharyngeus
120. Pharyngeal Constrictors

APPENDIX 4: TWO-JOINT MUSCLES

Biceps Brachii [20]
Biceps Femoris, Long Head [63]
Extensor Carpi Radialis Longus and Brevis [25]
Extensor Carpi Ulnaris [27]
Flexor Carpi Radialis [33]
Flexor Carpi Ulnaris [50]
Flexor Digitorum Superficialis [35]

Gastrocnemius [72]
Gracilis [59]
Palmaris Longus [34]
Rectus Femoris (of Quadriceps) [62]
Sartorius [61]
Semitendinosus and Semimembranosus [64]
Triceps Brachii [22]

APPENDIX 5: MUSCLES THAT HAVE DUAL INNERVATION

Adductor Magnus (Obturator, Sciatic) [57]
Biceps Femoris (Tibial, Peroneal) [63]
Brachialis (Musculocutaneous, Radial) [21]
Flexor Digitorum Profundus (Median, Ulnar) [37]
Flexor Pollicis Brevis (Median, Ulnar) [41]
Iliopsoas (L2-4, Femoral) [51]
Levator Palpebrae Superioris (CNIII, Sympathetic) [96]
Levator Scapulae (C3-4, "Occasionally" Dorsal Scapular) [5]
Levator Veli Palatini (CNX, CNXI) [113]
Lower Trapezius (CNXI, C2-4) [3]
Lumbricals (Median, Ulnar) [42]
Lumbricales (Medial and Lateral Plantar) [78]
Middle Trapezius (CNXI, C2-4) [2]

Omohyoid (Superior Ramus of Ansa Cervicalis and Ansa Cervicalis) [121]
Palatoglossus (CNIX, XI) [119]
Palatopharyngeus (CNXI, Pharyngeal Plexus) [115]
Pectineus (Femoral, Accessory Obturator when present) [58]
Pectoralis Major, Sternal Portion (Medial Pectoral, Lateral Pectoral) [10]
Salpingopharyngeus (CNX, CNXI) [114]
Sternocleidomastoid (CNXI, C2-3) [107]
Subscapularis (Upper Subscapular, Lower Subscapular) [16]
Upper Trapezius (CNXI, C2-4) [1]

APPENDIX 6: MUSCLES BY NERVE ROOT LEVEL

C1
Rectus Capitis Posterior Major and Minor
Obliquus Capitis Superior and Inferior

C2
Upper Trapezius
Middle Trapezius
Lower Trapezius
Rectus Capitis Posterior Major and Minor
Obliquus Capitis Superior and Inferior
Sternocleidomastoid

C3
Upper Trapezius
Middle Trapezius

Lower Trapezius
Levator Scapulae
Splenius Capitis and Cervicis
Sternocleidomastoid
Scalenus (Anterior, Medius, and Posterior)
Diaphragm

C4
Upper Trapezius
Middle Trapezius
Lower Trapezius
Levator Scapulae
Splenius Capitis and Cervicis
Scalenus (Anterior, Medius, and Posterior)
Diaphragm

C5
Rhomboid Major and Minor
Levator Scapulae
Serratus Anterior
Teres Major
Pectoralis Major, Clavicular Portion
Anterior Deltoid
Middle Deltoid
Posterior Deltoid
Teres Minor
Subscapularis
Supraspinatus
Infraspinatus
Coracobrachialis
Biceps Brachii
Brachialis
Brachioradialis
Supinator
Splenius Capitis and Cervicis
Scalenus (Anterior, Medius, and Posterior)
Diaphragm

C6
Serratus Anterior
Latissimus Dorsi
Teres Major
Pectoralis Major, Clavicular Portion
Anterior Deltoid
Middle Deltoid
Posterior Deltoid
Teres Minor
Subscapularis
Supraspinatus
Infraspinatus
Coracobrachialis
Biceps Brachii
Brachialis
Triceps Brachii and Anconeus
Brachioradialis
Supinator
Extensor Carpi Radialis Longus and Brevis
Extensor Digitorum Communis
Extensor Carpi Ulnaris
Extensor Indicis
Extensor Pollicis Longus
Abductor Pollicis Longus
Extensor Pollicis Brevis
Flexor Carpi Radialis
Pronator Teres
Splenius Capitis and Cervicis
Scalenus (Anterior, Medius, and Posterior)

C7
Serratus Anterior
Latissimus Dorsi
Pectoralis Major, Clavicular Portion
Pectoralis Minor

Coracobrachialis
Brachialis
Triceps Brachii and Anconeus
Extensor Carpi Radialis Longus and Brevis
Extensor Digitorum Communis
Extensor Carpi Ulnaris
Extensor Indicis
Extensor Pollicis Longus
Abductor Pollicis Longus
Extensor Pollicis Brevis
Flexor Carpi Radialis
Pronator Teres
Palmaris Longus
Flexor Digitorum Superficialis
Flexor Pollicis Longus
Flexor Digitorum Profundus
Pronator Quadratus
Abductor Pollicis Brevis
Opponens Pollicis
Flexor Pollicis Brevis, Deep and Superficial Heads
Lumbricals
Palmaris Brevis
Splenius Capitis and Cervicis
Scalenus (Anterior, Medius, and Posterior)

C8
Latissimus Dorsi
Pectoralis Major, Sternal Portion
Pectoralis Minor
Triceps Brachii and Anconeus
Extensor Digitorum Communis
Extensor Carpi Ulnaris
Extensor Indicis
Extensor Pollicis Longus
Abductor Pollicis Longus
Extensor Pollicis Brevis
Flexor Carpi Radialis
Palmaris Longus
Flexor Digitorum Superficialis
Flexor Pollicis Longus
Flexor Digitorum Profundus
Pronator Quadratus
Abductor Pollicis Brevis
Opponens Pollicis
Flexor Pollicis Brevis, Deep and Superficial Heads
Lumbricals
Palmaris Brevis
Opponens Digiti Minimi
Abductor Digiti Minimi
Flexor Digiti Minimi
Adductor Pollicis
Palmar Interossei
Dorsal Interossei
Flexor Carpi Ulnaris
Splenius Capitis and Cervicis
Scalenus (Anterior, Medius, and Posterior)

T1

Pectoralis Major, Sternal Portion
Pectoralis Minor
Palmaris Longus
Flexor Digitorum Superficialis
Flexor Pollicis Longus
Flexor Digitorum Profundus
Pronator Quadratus
Abductor Pollicis Brevis
Opponens Pollicis
Flexor Pollicis Brevis, Deep and Superficial
  Heads
Lumbricals
Palmaris Brevis
Opponens Digiti Minimi
Abductor Digiti Minimi
Flexor Digiti Minimi
Adductor Pollicis
Palmar Interossei
Dorsal Interossei
Flexor Carpi Ulnaris

T1-L2

Internal Intercostals (T1-11)
External Intercostals (T1-11)
Rectus Abdominis (T5-12)
External Oblique (T5-L1)
Internal Oblique (T5-L1)
Quadratus Lumborum (T12-L1)

L2

Iliopsoas
Adductor Brevis and Longus
Adductor Magnus
Pectineus
Gracilis
Sartorius
Quadriceps (Rectus Femoris, Vastus Lateralis, Medialis,
  and Intermedius)

L3

Iliopsoas
Adductor Brevis and Longus
Adductor Magnus
Pectineus
Gracilis
Sartorius
Quadriceps (Rectus Femoris, Vastus Lateralis, Medialis,
  and Intermedius)

L4

Iliopsoas
Gluteus Medius
Gluteus Minimus
Tensor Fascia Lata
Adductor Brevis and Longus
Adductor Magnus
Pectineus

Gracilis
Sartorius
Quadriceps (Rectus Femoris, Vastus Lateralis, Medialis,
  and Intermedius)
Popliteus
Tibialis Anterior
Extensor Digitorum Longus
Peroneus Tertius
Peroneii (Peroneus Longus and Brevis)

L5

Gluteus Maximus
Gluteus Medius
Gluteus Minimus
Tensor Fascia Lata
Adductor Magnus
Biceps Femoris (Short and Long Heads)
Semitendinosus and Semimembranosus
Popliteus
Tibialis Anterior
Extensor Digitorum Longus
Peroneus Tertius
Peroneii (Peroneus Longus and Brevis)
Extensor Hallucis Longus
Extensor Digitorum Brevis
Flexor Digitorum Longus
Tibialis Posterior
Gastrocnemius
Soleus
Flexor Hallucis Longus
Lumbricales (Foot)

S1

Gluteus Maximus
Gluteus Medius
Gluteus Minimus
Tensor Fascia Lata
Adductor Magnus
Piriformis
Biceps Femoris (Short and Long Heads)
Semitendinosus and Semimembranosus
Popliteus
Tibialis Anterior
Extensor Digitorum Longus
Peroneus Tertius
Peroneii (Peroneus Longus and Brevis)
Extensor Hallucis Longus
Extensor Digitorum Brevis
Flexor Digitorum Longus
Tibialis Posterior
Gastrocnemius
Soleus
Flexor Hallucis Longus
Lumbricales (Foot)
Abductor Hallucis
Plantar Interossei

Dorsal Interossei (Foot)
Abductor Digiti Minimi

S2
Gluteus Maximus
Piriformis
Biceps Femoris (Short and Long Heads)
Semitendinosus and Semimembranosus
Gastrocnemius
Soleus
Flexor Hallucis Longus
Lumbricales (Foot)
Abductor Hallucis
Plantar Interossei
Dorsal Interossei (Foot)
Abductor Digit Minimi

CNIII
Levator Palpebrae Superioris

CNV
Masseter
Temporalis
Median and Lateral Pterygoids
Tensor Veli Palatini
Mylohyoid
Digastric

CNVII
Frontalis
Nasalis
Procerus
Orbicularis Oculi
Orbicularis Oris
Zygomaticus Major and Minor
Buccinator
Platysma/Depressor Anguli Oris
Stylohyoid

CNIX
Stylopharyngeus
Palatoglossus

CNX
Levator Veli Palatini
Salpingopharyngeus

CNXI
Upper Trapezius
Middle Trapezius
Lower Trapezius
Sternocleidomastoid
Levator Veli Palatini
Salpingopharyngeus
Palatopharyngeus
Palatoglossus

CNXII
Geniohyoid
Tongue
Hyoglossus
Genioglossus
Styloglossus
Thyrohyoid

Ansa Cervicalis
Sternohyoid
Sternothyroid
Omohyoid

Sympathetic
Levator Palpebrae Superioris

Pharyngeal Plexus
Palatopharyngeus
Pharyngeal Constrictors

Dorsal Rami of Corresponding Levels
Iliocostalis Cervicis, Thoracis, and Lumborum
Longissimus Capitis, Cervicis, and Thoracis
Spinalis Capitis, Cervicis, and Thoracis
Semispinalis Capitis and Cervicis
Multifidus
Rotatores

APPENDIX 7: MUSCLES LISTED BY CHAPTER

CHAPTER 3: SHOULDER AND ARM AND UPPER BACK

Spinal Accessory
1. Upper Trapezius (CNXI, C2-4)
2. Middle Trapezius (CNXI, C2-4)
3. Lower Trapezius (CNXI, C2-4)

Dorsal Scapular
4. Rhomboid Major and Minor (C5)
5. Levator Scapulae (C3-5)

Long Thoracic
6. Serratus Anterior (C5-7)

Thoracodorsal
7. Latissimus Dorsi (C6-8)

Lower Subscapular
8. Teres Major (C5-6)

Lateral Pectoral
9. Pectoralis Major Clavicular Portion (C5-7)

Medial and Lateral Pectoral
10. Pectoralis Major Sternal Portion (C8-T1)

Medial Pectoral
11. Pectoralis Minor (C7-T1)

Axillary
12. Anterior Deltoid (C5-6)
13. Middle Deltoid (C5-6)
14. Posterior Deltoid (C5-6)
15. Teres Minor (C5-6)

Upper and Lower Subscapular
16. Subscapularis (C5-6)

Suprascapular
17. Supraspinatus (C5-6)
18. Infraspinatus (C5-6)

Musculocutaneous
19. Coracobrachialsis (C5-7)
20. Biceps Brachii (C5-6)
21. Brachialis (C5-7)

Radial
21. Brachialis (C5-7)
22. Triceps Brachii and Anconeus (C6-8)

CHAPTER 4: FOREARM AND HAND

Radial
23. Brachioradialis (C5-6)
24. Supinator (C5-6)
25. Extensor Carpi Radialis Longus and Brevis (C6-7)
26. Extensor Digitorum Communis (C6-8)
27. Extensor Carpi Ulnaris (C6-8)
28. Extensor Indicis (C6-8)
29. Extensor Pollicis Longus (C6-8)
30. Abductor Pollicis Longus (C6-8)
31. Extensor Pollicis Brevis (C6-8)

Median
32. Pronator Teres (C6-7)
33. Flexor Carpi Radialis (C6-8)
34. Palmaris Longus (C7-T1)
35. Flexor Digitorum Superficialis (C7-T1)
36. Flexor Pollicis Longus (C7-T1)
37. Flexor Digitorum Profundus (and Ulnar) (C7-T1)
38. Pronator Quadratus (C7-T1)
39. Abductor Pollicis Brevis (C7-T1)
40. Opponens Pollicis (C7-T1)
41. Flexor Pollicis Brevis: Deep and Superficial Heads (and Ulnar) (C7-T1)
42. Lumbricals (and Ulnar) (C7-T1)

Ulnar
43. Opponens Digiti Minimi (C8-T1)
44. Abductor Digiti Minimi (C8-T1)
45. Flexor Digiti Minimi (C8-T1)
46. Adductor Pollicis (C8-T1)
47. Palmar Interossei (C8-T1)
48. Dorsal Interossei (C8-T1)
49. Palmaris Brevis (C7-T1)
37. Flexor Digitorum Profundus (and Median) (C7-T1)
41. Flexor Pollicis Brevis: Deep and Superficial Heads (and Median) (C7-T1)

42. Lumbricals (and Median) (C7-T1)
50. Flexor Carpi Ulnaris (C8-T1)

CHAPTER 5: HIP AND THIGH

Lumbar Roots and Femoral
51. Iliopsoas (L2-4)

Inferior Gluteal
52. Gluteus Maximus (L5-S2)

Superior Gluteal
53. Gluteus Medius (L4-S1)
54. Gluteus Minimus (L4-S1)
55. Tensor Fascia Lata (L4-S1)

Obturator
56. Adductor Brevis and Longus (L2-4)
57. Adductor Magnus (and Sciatic) (L2-S1)
58. Pectineus (L2-4)
59. Gracilis (L2-4)

Sacral Plexus
60. Hip Rotators (Piriformis) (S1-2)

Femoral
61. Sartorius (L2-4)
62. Quadriceps (Rectus Femoris, Vastus Lateralis, Medialis, and Intermedius) (L2-4)

Sciatic (Tibial and Peroneal Divisions)
63. Biceps Femoris (Short and Long Heads) (L5-S2)
64. Semitendinosus and Semimembranosus (L5-S2)

Tibial
65. Popliteus (L4-S1)

CHAPTER 6: LEG AND FOOT

Deep Peroneal
66. Tibialis Anterior (L4-S1)
67. Extensor Digitorum Longus (L4-S1)
68. Extensor Hallucis Longus (L5-S1)
69. Peroneus Tertius (L4-S1)
70. Extensor Digitorum Brevis (L5-S1)

Superficial Peroneal
71. Peroneii (Peroneus Longus and Brevis) (L4-S1)

Tibial
72. Gastrocnemius (L5-S2)
73. Soleus (L5-S2)
74. Flexor Digitorum Longus (L5-S1)
75. Flexor Hallucis Longus (L5-S2)
76. Tibialis Posterior (L5-S1)

Plantars
77. Abductor Hallucis (S1-2)
78. Lumbricales (L5-S2)
79. Plantar Interossei (S1-2)
80. Dorsal Interossei (S1-2)
81. Abductor Digiti Minimi (S1-2)

CHAPTER 7: TRUNK AND PARASPINALS

Ventral Roots
82. Rectus Abdominis (T5-T12)
83. External Oblique (T5-L1)
84. Internal Oblique (T5-L1)
85. Quadratus Lumborum (T12-L1)

Dorsal Roots
86. Iliocostalis Cervicis, Thoracis, and Lumborum
87. Longissimus Capitis, Cervicis, and Thoracis
88. Spinalis Capitis, Cervicis, and Thoracis
89. Semispinalis Capitis and Cervicis
90. Multifidus
91. Rotatores

CHAPTER 8: HEAD NECK AND FACE
92. Frontalis (CNVII)
93. Nasalis (CNVII)
94. Procerus (CNVII)
95. Orbicularis Oculi (CNVII)
96. Levator Palpebrae Superioris (CNIII, Sympathetic)
97. Orbicularis Oris (CNVII)
98. Zygomaticus Major and Minor (CNVII)
99. Buccinator (CNVII)
100. Platysma / Depressor Anguli Oris (CNVII)
101. Masseter (CNV)
102. Temporalis (CNV)
103. Medial and Lateral Pterygoids (CNV)
104. Splenius Capitis and Cervicis (Dorsal Rami C3-8)
105. Rectus Capitis Posterior Major and Minor (Dorsal Rami C1-2)
106. Obliquus Capitis Superior and Inferior (Dorsal Rami C1-2)
107. Sternocleidomastoid (CNXI, C2-3)
108. Scalenus (Anterior, Medius, and Posterior) (Ventral Rami C3-8)

CHAPTER 9: MUSCLES OF RESPIRATION

Phrenic
109. Diaphragm (C3-5)

Intercostals
110. External Intercostals (T1-11)
111. Internal Intercostals (T1 11)

CHAPTER 10: SWALLOWING
112. Tensor Veli Palatini (CNV)
113. Levator Veli Palatini (CNX, XI)
114. Salpingopharyngeus (CNX, XI)
115. Palatopharyngeus (CNXI, Pharyngeal Plexus)
116. Stylopharyngeus (CNIX)
117. Geniohyoid (CNXII), Mylohyoid (CNV), Stylohyoid (CNVII), Digastric (CNV)
118. Tongue (CNXII)
119. Tongue Extrinsic Muscles: Hyoglossus (CNXII), Genioglossus (CNXII), Styloglossus (CNXII), Palatoglossus (CNIX, XI)
120. Pharyngeal Constrictors (Pharyngeal Plexus)
121. Infrahyoid Muscles: Sternohyoid (Ansa Cervicalis), Sternothyroid (Ansa Cervicalis), Omohyoid (Superior Ramus of Ansa Cervicalis and Ansa Cervicalis), Thyrohyoid (CNXII)

APPENDIX 8: MUSCLES BY FUNCTION

SHOULDER FLEXION
Anterior Deltoid [12]
Coracobrachialis [19]
Long Head of Biceps Brachii [20]
Pectoralis Major (Clavicular) [9]

SHOULDER EXTENSION
Latissimus Dorsi [7]
Teres Major [8]
Posterior Deltoid [14]
Long Head of Triceps Brachii [22]
Pectoralis Major (when the shoulder is flexed beyond 90 degrees) [9,10]

SHOULDER ABDUCTION
Anterior Deltoid (in combination with the Posterior Deltoid) [12]
Middle Deltoid [13]
Supraspinatus [17]
Biceps Brachii (in combination with other abductors when the shoulder is abducted beyond 90 degrees) [20]

SHOULDER ADDUCTION
Latissimus Dorsi [7]
Teres Major [8]
Pectoralis Major (Clavicular) [9]
Pectoralis Major (Sternal) [10]
Coracobrachialis [19]
Long Head of Triceps Brachii [22]

SHOULDER HORIZONTAL ADDUCTION
Pectoralis Major (Clavicular) [9]
Anterior Deltoid [12]
Coracobrachialis [19]

SHOULDER HORIZONTAL ABDUCTION
Posterior Deltoid [14]

SHOULDER INTERNAL ROTATION
Latissimus Dorsi [7]
Teres Major [8]
Pectoralis Major (Clavicular) [9]
Anterior Deltoid [12]
Subscapularis [16]

SHOULDER EXTERNAL ROTATION
Posterior Deltoid [14]
Teres Minor [15]
Infraspinatus [18]

ELBOW FLEXION
Biceps Brachii [20]
Brachialis [21]
Brachioradialis [23]
Pronator Teres [32]
Extensor Carpi Radialis Longus [25]
Flexor Carpi Radialis [33]
Palmaris Longus [34]
Flexor Carpi Ulnaris [50]

ELBOW EXTENSION
Triceps Brachii [22]
Anconeus [22]

FOREARM SUPINATION
Biceps Brachii [20]
Brachioradialis [23]
Supinator [24]

FOREARM PRONATION
Brachioradialis [23]
Pronator Teres [32]
Pronator Quadratus [38]
Flexor Carpi Radialis [33]

WRIST EXTENSION
Extensor Carpi Radialis Longus [25]
Extensor Carpi Radialis Brevis [25]
Extensor Carpi Ulnaris [27]
Extensor Digitorum Communis [26]
Extensor Indicis [28]
Extensor Pollicis Longus [29]

WRIST FLEXION
Flexor Carpi Radialis [33]
Flexor Carpi Ulnaris [50]
Palmaris Longus [34]
Flexor Digitorum Profundus [37]
Flexor Digitorum Superficialis [35]
Flexor Pollicis Longus [36]

WRIST ULNAR DEVIATION
Flexor Carpi Ulnaris [50]
Extensor Carpi Ulnaris [27]

WRIST RADIAL DEVIATION
Flexor Carpi Radialis [33]
Extensor Carpi Radialis Longus [25]
Extensor Carpi Radialis Brevis [25]
Extensor Pollicis Longus [29]
Extensor Pollicis Brevis [31]
Abductor Pollicis Longus [30]

METACARPOPHALANGEAL JOINT FLEXION
Dorsal Interossei [48]
Palmar Interossei [47]
Abductor Digiti Minimi [44]
Flexor Digiti Minimi [45]
Flexor Pollicis Longus [36]
Flexor Pollicis Brevis [41]
Flexor Digitorum Profundus [37]
Flexor Digitorum Superficialis [35]
Adductor Pollicis [46]

INTERPHALANGEAL JOINT FLEXION
Flexor Digitorum Profundus [37]
Flexor Digitorum Superficialis [35]
Flexor Pollicis Longus [36]

METACARPOPHALANGEAL JOINT EXTENSION
Extensor Digitorum Communis [26]
Extensor Indicis [28]
Extensor Pollicis Longus [29]
Extensor Pollicis Brevis [31]

INTERPHALANGEAL JOINT EXTENSION
Lumbricals [42]
Dorsal Interossei [48]
Palmar Interossei [47]
Extensor Digitorum Communis [26]
Extensor Indicis [28]
Extensor Pollicis Longus [29]

THUMB CARPOMETACARPAL JOINT FLEXION
Flexor Pollicis Longus [36]
Flexor Pollicis Brevis [41]
Opponens Pollicis [40]

THUMB INTERPHALANGEAL JOINT FLEXION
Flexor Pollicis Longus [36]

THUMB CARPOMETACARPAL JOINT EXTENSION
Extensor Pollicis Longus [29]
Abductor Pollicis Longus [30]
Extensor Pollicis Brevis [31]

THUMB INTERPHALANGEAL JOINT EXTENSION
Extensor Pollicis Longus [29]
Abductor Pollicis Brevis [39]

THUMB CARPOMETACARPAL ABDUCTION
Abductor Pollicis Brevis [39]
Abductor Pollicis Longus [30]
Extensor Pollicis Brevis [31]

THUMB CARPOMETACARPAL ADDUCTION
Adductor Pollicis [46]

THUMB CARPOMETACARPAL OPPOSITION
Opponens Pollicis [40]
Abductor Pollicis Brevis [39]
Flexor Pollicis Brevis [41]

HIP FLEXION
Iliopsoas [51]
Quadriceps (Rectus Femoris) [62]
Pectineus [58]
Tensor Fascia Lata [55]
Gluteus Minimus [54]
Sartorius [61]
Adductor Longus [56]
Adductor Magnus (Anterior Part) [57]
Adductor Brevis [56]
Gluteus Medius [53]

HIP EXTENSION
Gluteus Maximus [52]
Adductor Magnus (Posterior Part) [57]
Piriformis [60]
Semimembranosus [64]
Semitendinosus [64]
Gluteus Medius [53]
Biceps Femoris (Long Head) [63]

HIP ABDUCTION
Gluteus Medius [53]
Gluteus Minimus [54]
Gluteus Maximus (can assist in abduction when the hip is flexed) [52]
Sartorius [61]
Tensor Fascia Lata [55]
Piriformis [60]

HIP ADDUCTION
Adductor Brevis [56]
Pectineus [58]
Adductor Magnus [57]
Gracilis [59]
Gluteus Maximus [52]
Adductor Longus [56]
Iliopsoas [51]

HIP INTERNAL ROTATION
Gluteus Medius [53]
Gluteus Minimis [54]
Tensor Fascia Lata [55]
Semitendinosus [64]
Semimembranosus [64]

HIP EXTERNAL ROTATION
Gluteus Maximus [52]
Sartorius [61]

Piriformis [60] (as well as other small external rotator muscles of the hip, not mentioned in this book)
Gluteus Medius [53]
Iliopsoas [51]
Biceps Femoris (Long Head) [63]

KNEE FLEXION
Semitendinosus [64]
Semimembranosus [64]
Biceps Femoris [63]
Gracilis [59]
Sartorius [61]
Gastrocnemius [72]
Poplietus [65]
Tensor Fascia Lata [55]

KNEE EXTENSION
Quadriceps Femoris [62]
Gluteus Maximus (via iliotibial band) [52]

KNEE INTERNAL ROTATION
Semitendinosus [64]
Semimembranosis [64]
Popliteus [65]
Gracilis [59]
Sartorius [61]

KNEE EXTERNAL ROTATION
Biceps Femoris [63]

ANKLE DORSIFLEXION
Tibialis Anterior [66]
Peroneus Tertius [69]
Extensor Hallucis Longus [68]
Extensor Digitorum Longus [67]

ANKLE PLANTARFLEXION
Gastrocnemius [72]
Soleus [73]
Flexor Digitorum Longus [74]
Flexor Hallucis Longus [75]
Tibialis Posterior [76]
Peroneus Longus and Brevis [71]

INVERSION
Tibialis Anterior [66]
Tibialis Posterior [76]
Flexor Digitorum Longus [74]
Flexor Hallucis Longus [75]
Extensor Hallucis Longus [68]
Gastrocnemius (via the Achilles tendon) [72]
Soleus (via the Achilles tendon) [73]

EVERSION
Peroneus Longus and Brevis [71]
Peroneus Tertius [69]
Extensor Digitorum Longus [67]

TOE FLEXION
Flexor Digitorum Longus [74]
Lumbricales [78]

Dorsal Interossei [80]
Plantar Interossei [79]

TOE EXTENSION
Extensor Digitorum Longus [67]
Extensor Digitorum Brevis [70]

GREAT TOE FLEXION
Flexor Hallucis Longus [75]
Abductor Hallucis [77]

GREAT TOE EXTENSION
Extensor Hallucis Longus [68]
Extension Digitorum Brevis [70]

MASTICATION
Medial Pterygoid [103]
Lateral Pterygoid [103]
Temporalis [102]
Masseter [101]

JAW CLOSING
Medial Pterygoid [103]
Temporalis [102]
Masseter [101]

JAW OPENING
Lateral Pteryoid [103]

SMILING
Zygomaticus Major [98]
Zygomaticus Minor [98]
Buccinator [99]
Risorius

FROWNING
Platysma [100]
Depressor Anguli Oris [100]

APPENDIX 9: MUSCLES OMITTED FROM THIS BOOK

Anterior Vertebral Muscles (Longus Cervicis, Capitis,
    Rectus Capitis Ant, Lateral,)
Corrugator Supercilii
Depressor Septi
Levator Angular Oris
Risorius
Levator Labi Superioris
Mentalis
Extensor Digiti Minimi
Subclavius
Gemellus Inferior
Gemellus Superior

Obturator Internus
Obturator Externus
Quadratus Femoris
Extensor Hallucis Brevis
Flexor Hallucis Brevis
Flexor Digiti Minimi Brevis
Flexor Digitorum Brevis
Quadratus Planti
Abductor Digiti Minimi
Adductor Hallucis
Intertransverseii

INDEX

ISBN 0-07-033150-2

90000

9 780070 331501